5-2011
amazon
$37.00

☞ W9-BLM-639

Cancer-Free

Your Guide to Gentle, Non-toxic Healing
[Third Edition]

By

Bill Henderson

616.994
HEN

ARCADIA PUBLIC LIBRARY
ARCADIA, WI 54612

Copyright © 2008 Bill Henderson

ISBN-13 978-1-60145-183-5
ISBN-10 1-60145-183-0

All rights reserved. No part of this publication may be reproduced, stored in a
retrieval system, or transmitted in any form or by any means, electronic,
mechanical, recording or otherwise, without the prior written permission of the
author.

Printed in the United States of America.

Booklocker.com, Inc.
2008

Previous books by this author:

Cure Your Cancer (e-book), published November 2000

Cure Your Cancer (paperback and hard cover) published by
AuthorHouse, Inc., June 2003

Cancer-Free (paperback and e-book) [First Edition] published by
Son-Rise Publications, November 2004

Cancer-Free (paperback and e-book) (Second Edition)
published by Booklocker, Inc., June, 2007

Web Site: http://www.Beating-Cancer-Gently.com

DISCLAIMER

This book details the author's personal experiences with and opinions about cancer. Neither the author nor the publisher is a healthcare provider.

The author and publisher are providing this book and its contents on an "as is" basis and make no representations or warranties of any kind with respect to this book or its contents. The author and publisher disclaim all such representations and warranties, including for example warranties of merchantability and healthcare for a particular purpose. In addition, the author and publisher do not represent or warrant that the information accessible via this book is accurate, complete or current.

The statements made about products and services have not been evaluated by the U.S. Food and Drug Administration. They are not intended to diagnose, treat, cure, or prevent any condition or disease. Please consult with your own physician or healthcare specialist regarding the suggestions and recommendations made in this book.

Except as specifically stated in this book, neither the author or publisher, nor any authors, contributors, or other representatives will be liable for damages arising out of or in connection with the use of this book. This is a comprehensive limitation of liability that applies to all damages of any kind, including (without limitation) compensatory; direct, indirect or consequential damages; loss of data, income or profit; loss of or damage to property and claims of third parties.

You understand that this book is not intended as a substitute for consultation with a licensed healthcare practitioner, such as your physician. Before you begin any healthcare program, or change your lifestyle in any way, you will consult your physician or other licensed healthcare practitioner to ensure that you are in good health and that the examples contained in this book will not harm you.

This book provides content related to topics concerning physical and/or mental health issues. As such, use of this book implies your acceptance of this disclaimer.

READERS' FEEDBACK....

Greetings! I am ecstatic! They can't find any more cancer after telling me I was a Stage IV – terminal last July. It was recurrent breast cancer from 15 years ago which showed up in fluid in a sac in the lung. I talked to you in August and started your plan. I did not cheat one crumb – I was religious about all of it. By the end of September, that was all clear. My scans last week were great – no activity anywhere that they could find and the doctor was STUNNED. I have been asked to speak before a breast cancer support group this Thursday night, so you might be contacted for more books. Life is good -- God is wonderful. He has helped me find these healing things and I thank him for all of you out there who want to help people. My e-mail is full and my phone has been busy with people calling wanting to know what I did. But it is a good feeling.

Thank you, thank you, thank you – what a blessing.

Sandra Goldberg
Little Rock, Arkansas

I have purchased two of your books, Cancer-Free, and find them outstanding publications. There are no other books, or help, on the subject of Cancer out there to match, or even come close to yours. I truly hope you find a major publisher to help you. I really enjoy your newsletters and have forwarded them to many, many people. God bless you.

J.M. Larmer, Naturopathic Doctor
New Jersey

Hi Bill, I am a nurse...I found your website by chance when a life long friend called me over a year ago to tell me he had liver cancer. The survival rate for this type of cancer is very poor. You were an answer to a prayer.

He started on MGN-3 right away and shared your book with his oncologist. His cancer went into remission within a couple of months and he is cancer free now. Thank you.

I share the information about your research. My own father died two years ago on January 16, 2001 of esophageal cancer that metastasized to his lungs. From the time his cancer was diagnosed until he died was less than two months. I only wish I had known about you and your book sooner.

I don't want others to lose their loved ones before their time if I can help by telling them about your book. May God bless you Bill. Thank you.

Faye Maier
North Carolina

Hi Bill, Went back for CT scans September 25th – exactly one year + one day from the day they told me I had Cancer in my stomach, lung and adrenal gland. Guess what!! Lung cancer is gone and the other two have not grown!!! Praise God! All this because my granddaughter found your site while looking for help. God does work in mysterious ways. I am still pain-free, thank God!!! And doing well...I have you to thank for finding out about Protocel. I wish there was a way to tell the World!!! Thank you, again.

Libby

Dear Bill, Thank you for your excellent book. It is very informative and will help me in my search for the best combination of treatments there are for patients…the book is wonderful, informative and very accurate.

Dr. Dana Flavin (cancer doctor)
Connecticut, USA

Dear Mr. Henderson and readers:

My name is Dr. Tom. I have watched my significant other follow the advice of oncologists for over a year to find that their advice is ill conceived. I watched resident medical doctors follow their mentor, a head oncologist, into the blinded view of chemotherapy treatment for cancer patients. To watch this is clearly an eye opener on how brain washed medical doctors are. Like puppets following the puppet master into the show on stage. The horrifying truth of it all is that people trust and believe in these prescription drug pushers.

To understand the background of how corrupt the oncology system is, one must get the background of how corrupt the medical establishment is. The book Politics In Healing is a good read for starters. The largest, most traditional cancer treatment centers are the most criminal; and the young doctors are clueless to this being the case, since they are only told what they need to know to push the chemotherapeutic agents on cancer patients who later become the oncologists' victims. Now that the media is starting to notice this, I will speak it more freely.

What the public doesn't know is that the reason why some people get cured of cancer while on chemotherapy is not because chemotherapy works, but because alternative treatment works and chemotherapy slows down the curing and makes it more difficult for the alternative treatment to work. What I want to get across is that traditional medical treatment for cancer is worse than ineffective and that any change of lifestyle without chemotherapy would be more effective in reducing the cancer than chemotherapy.

Sincerely,

Dr. T.
Virginia, USA

This book helped save my Mother's life.

With a whole world of information out there on the Internet about cancer it can leave you confused and feel like you are running around in a maze not knowing where to turn or what to believe. This book helped me get informed and ready to help my mother in just a few hours.

I found Bill Henderson's book to be an excellent overview of numerous natural treatments for cancer. He is not selling any product or promoting a single treatment method. Instead I found the book to be an extremely well written, intelligent, concise and to the point overview of many excellent natural cancer treatments. Also included are treatments that will help people already on chemotherapy.

The book allows you to track down more information about your favorite treatment by providing website addresses and suggests where you can get natural products at the cheapest prices (in the USA). It really helps the reader to be fully informed about ALL their options other than just surgery, radiation or chemotherapy.

The testimonials were very convincing and helped me to have the confidence to help my mother who was near death

(suffering from advanced metastatic breast cancer that has spread to the liver, lungs, ovaries and bones) to keep taking dried barley greens. Within 2 days her strong pain levels had improved. After 9 days she was COMPLETELY off all pain and nausea medication and in NO PAIN whatsoever. I am so thankful I read this book and became more informed about the many, well known, tried and proven natural treatments out there. Thank you, Bill Henderson.

Peter Mita

Melbourne, Australia

If you love your stricken one, this is your "Bible."

Denzel Koh
Brisbane, Australia

Bill, you do a great service. I have directed a number of people to you, and all of them say the same thing. Keep going, Bill, and if I can help you any way, you have my e-mail address.

Herb
Dr. Herb Tabor
http://www.drtabor.healingamerica.com/

Hi Bill: Thanks much for your guidance and advice. You are doing a great deed for humanity. By way of recognition, I must report to you great results we had through your recommendations. Based on your advice we started using Dr. Budwig's diet fo/cc + red raspberries, MGN-3, co-Q10, Wobenzyme. She had 4 treatments with chemo all the time complementing it with the above regimen. Today I'm happy to report that we did a full body PET/CT scan the results came back: A complete resolution in the left breast, no lymphatic involvement, an 80% reduction in the manubrium uptake. Quite dramatic to the amazement of my oncologist who told me he did recommend this regimen to other patients, even some of his family members. It also helped her to minimize the side effects of chemo. Throughout the whole time, she never missed a day of work except the day of the treatment.

Thanks a Million
Simon

Dear Bill, I want to thank YOU for all of the hard work and dedication that you've put into this labor of love!!! I truly appreciate all of this information Bill, and I consider it truly a blessing from God that I stumbled across the link to your website. My Mom has Acute Lymphocytic Leukemia, but she is currently in remission...I want to thank you from the bottom of my heart!

Natasha

God will take you into the Palm of his Hand Bill. You are an amazing person. And your next life will reflect what you have done in this one.

Blessings, and thank you.

Anne Mozdzanowski
Denmark

Hi, Bill. Got a copy of your book not more than a week ago. I've been working on a dissertation for a second PhD on alternative therapy for cancer. I'm sure I will be quoting you (and giving credit where credit is due, of course) in my research. Your book is well written, makes no absurd promises, and indeed offers hope. As a registered nurse, I

have become increasingly disillusioned by the "miracle of modern medicine" in connection with the treatment of cancers. We have NOT improved the lives of anyone. Chemo and radiation patients usually succumb to another devastating illness because of the lack of immune response. The medical community fails to give these details to the patient.

Dr. Randy Walden, RN, Ph.D.

Dear Bill,

Thanks to your many years of selflessness, you correctly say that the information in your archives is timeless and therefore of eternal use. Much of what you have communicated is supported by age-old wisdom, which further proves the timelessness of your massive and well-documented contribution.

Thank you for your ongoing dedication to helping people eradicate their bodily reactions. I know without any doubt that that's what it is, as the longer I pursue my 75% raw vegan diet the harder it becomes to detect a lump that was very palpable three years ago (there is probably no more than 10% of it left and I rarely if ever bother to feel for it anymore as it's no longer easy to find !).

I'd also like to thank you for the extreme lucidity and quality of the communication in your Newsletters. You are a very strong exponent of the English language and nothing of what you say is ever ambiguous or confusing. It is often obvious that you've gone to great lengths to ensure this and it's a sure sign of dedication to your readers. Thanks for being so particular - it contributes greatly to the timeless value of your Newsletters as they always reveal something new or make something that we've already read some time back appear clearer whenever one dips back into them. Your "drastic" and "permanent" guidance is one such example, and just look at the effect it's had on me!

God bless you always.

Kind regards,

Gary Gillespie, Great Britain

PREFACE

Hi. My name is Bill Henderson. In November 1990, my former wife, Marjorie, began her four-year bout with cancer. She died on November 1, 1994. Her many operations, chemotherapy treatments and intense pain made her wish often in her last two years for a quick death, or "transition," as she called it.

After watching that, it was hard for me to believe that millions of people each year had to endure that same torture. I have read widely since 1994, looking for options we were ignorant about. I have found over three hundred!

Realizing that millions of cancer patients needed this information to survive, I began what has become my full-time crusade. In books, newsletters, workshops, telephone coaching and a weekly radio show, I have tried to reach as many people as I can with this life-saving message.

I spend every day talking by e-mail and telephone with cancer patients. I am not a doctor. I am just a "reporter." However, with the information I have gathered, I have been able to help thousands of people all over the world become cancer-free. The only thing I sell is this book. My newsletters and radio shows are free.

If you haven't signed up for my newsletter, please do so now. Just go to my web site: www.Beating-Cancer-Gently.com and enter your name and e-mail address. My newsletters, which I publish once a month, are designed to update the information in this book. Over 15,000 readers in 71 countries receive this newsletter now. While at my web site, you may want to read some of the newsletter articles. Just click on the "Newsletter Archive" link.

In a previous book called "Cure Your Cancer" and the earlier version of this book, I reached about 8,000 cancer patients in 54 countries. I have been interviewed on 45 radio shows. I have presented dozens of workshops around the U.S. on "Beating Cancer – Gently." I have conducted 16 telephone conference calls on the same subject. Since October, 2007, I have hosted a web talk radio show called "How to Live Cancer-Free." Over 50,000 people listen each week. -You will find it at: http://www.WebTalkRadio.net

Now I want to help YOU. If this book can convince you how vital it is to take charge of your own health care, I will be delighted. Because then becoming cancer-free is just a matter of time.

Once you have made that crucial decision to "become smarter than your oncologist," there are literally hundreds of options – doctors, clinics, supplements, diet changes, detoxification methods – that will get you cancer-free. This book boils them down to a simple, six-part regimen which anyone can do and anyone can afford. It has worked to free hundreds of people of their cancer since November, 2004, when the first edition of this book was published.

The major difference between now and 1990-1994, when I was searching for information to help Marjorie, is the Internet. Now cancer patients have, as Hawaiians would say, a "tsunami" ("tidal wave" to us "haoles") of information on over 300 gentle, non-toxic treatments. My recommended regimen in Chapter 5 of this book is six of those 300 – and it works. I explain why to you in Chapter 5. It's no accident.

In this book, you have the benefit of eight years of feedback I have received from a vibrant network of doctors, nutritionists, cancer survivors and crusaders like me. People like Bob Davis, George Freaner, Art Brown, Gavin Phillips, Tony Preston, Webster Kehr, Michael Vrentas, Paul Winter, Dr. Mike Thompson, Dr. Ron Wheeler, Herb Horky, Ed VanOverloop, Dr. John Tate, Roger DeLong, Dr. Ralph Moss, Fred Eichhorn, Dr. Joseph Mercola, Dr. David Gregg, Dr. Richard Kinsolving, Dr. Loretta Lanphier, Ann Fonfa, Dr. Vincent Gammill, Dr. Dana Flavin and many more have all helped explode my knowledge with their personal assistance.

Authors I have discovered since my first book was published include Daniel Haley and his wonderful book "Politics in Healing;" T. Colin Campbell, Ph.D. and his interesting book on nutrition "The China Study," Jon Barron's "Lessons From The Miracle Doctors;" Les Winick's "The Reference Guide For Prostate Cancer, " Roger Mason's "The Natural Prostate Cure," Dr. Matthias Rath and his unique book "Cancer," Dr. Ralph Moss and his 13 books on cancer, Anne Frahm's book "A Cancer Battle Plan" and Ty Bollinger's "Cancer – Step Outside The Box." There are many more that will be mentioned in this text, but you get the idea. The resources available to you are incredibly rich.

Finally, organizations and non-commercial websites abound now to help you in your quest for perfect health. They include: CancerTutor.com; AlternativeMedicine.us; The American College for Advancement in Medicine; The Life Extension Foundation; The National Foundation For Alternative Medicine; The Cancer Control Society; The Health Sciences Institute; The National Cancer Research Foundation; The Cancer Cure Foundation; People Against Cancer; The Foundation For The Advancement of Innovative Medicine; Health Sciences Institute; and The American Biological Dentist Association.

I mention all of these only to impress you with the vast array of support available to you now. Believe me, nothing like this was available in 1994 when Marge and I needed it. Most of these people and organizations have web sites and newsletters that are extremely helpful in finding the right products and people to help you. Just like me, caring and not money motivates them.

My background is in computer software and marketing. After retiring from the U.S. Air Force as a Colonel in 1977, I founded a software publishing company that sold specialized software to architects and engineers. It was the first of its kind in the world. We had clients in 42 states and 4 Canadian provinces. I sold that company in 1995.

In addition to my medical research and writing, I have tried several other Internet ventures. I have a Masters in Business Administration from George Washington University. I am an entrepreneur at heart.

This book, however, is a true labor of love. I know how much it can help you, if you will trust me and keep an open mind. I was 76 in January 2008. My family and I have probably dealt with over 200 doctors and at least 10 of them have been close friends. When I lived in San Antonio, I played golf twice a week with a pediatrician, who is my best friend. In the last few years, I have had several encounters with the medical system.

In 1992, I met Joe Davis, M.D. He started me on a workout plan that I have continued ever since. He also convinced me of the importance of proper nutrition. He founded several "fitness centers" called Ultra-Fit in San Antonio. Bonus Booklet #2, "Stop Your Aging With Exercise," will summarize Dr. Davis' contribution to my current health.

In 1996, I had radial keratotomy done on one eye and laser correction on the other, which has allowed me to abandon the glasses I had worn all my life. I now wear glasses only for reading and computer work. In 1997, I had torn retinas repaired in both eyes. My vision is better now than ever before in my life. I had a hernia in my groin repaired very professionally in 1998. I had my sinuses cleaned out in 1999, which completely cured my chronic sinusitis. The doctor said she stopped counting when she got to 104 polyps removed.

Like most men my age, I have an enlarged prostate gland. Two urologists have treated me for the last 20 years. In a span of fourteen years, they did four biopsies on my prostate, all of which were negative. If I had known what I know now, I would not have had those biopsies done.

I feel much better physically now in every way than I did forty years ago. I mention my recent medical experience only to emphasize to you that I am anything but anti-doctor. Medical doctors serve a fine purpose in our society. If I had a trauma or other medical crisis, I would trust most American doctors to give me the finest care possible. However, their view of the treatment of cancer and other degenerative conditions is obscured by the bias in our society caused by the huge amount of money and its influence wielded by the pharmaceutical companies ("Big Pharma").

You have received with this "Cancer-Free" book four additional "booklets." They are at the end of this book under the same cover. Their titles are:

"Stop Your Aging With Diet"
"Stop Your Aging With Exercise"
"Beating Diabetes"
and "Cure Your Back Pain"

I have avoided using footnotes in this book. It is not a scholarly work for researchers. It is a "how-to" book for people with cancer or who have relatives or friends with cancer. The sources I have used can be found in Appendix A, along with a list of many other resources.

Before you read this book, I must give you the following warning and disclaimer:

The author of this book is a researcher and writer, not a physician. The facts presented in the following pages are offered as information only, not medical advice. Their purpose is to create the basis for informed consent. Although there is much that each of us can do in the area of prevention, self-treatment for clinical cancer, diabetes and back problems is not advised. The administration of therapy for these maladies, including nutritional therapy, should be under the supervision of health-care professionals who are specialists in their fields.

TABLE OF CONTENTS

CHAPTER 1
INTRODUCTION – WINNING THE CANCER WAR

"Nature makes the cure; the doctor's job is to aid nature."
Hippocrates (400 B.C.)

I am **honored** with the prospect of being able to help you treat your cancer or that of your loved one. In the ten years I have been counseling people on how to cope with cancer, they have taught me that the **only three reasons** people die of cancer today are: 1] lack of information; 2] lack of discipline once they have the information; and 3] blind trust in their cancer doctors.

The word cancer in your diagnosis **always** creates fear. This is part of the culture we live in. The fear of disability and pain is actually greater than the fear of death. Let me tell you something you can absolutely rely on. No cancer diagnosis is **a death notice**.

Why Listen To Me?

You have two choices. Seek out information on your own like what is in this book or listen to your doctors. I urge you to read for 10 to 20 hours (including the rest of this book) to become **"smarter than your oncologist"** about cancer. Really. That's all it takes.

Cancer is the **easiest** of the degenerative conditions to reverse. Much easier than diabetes, for example. Once you understand what cancer is, the way it is treated by cancer doctors **makes no sense.**

I'm not selling anything except this book. None of the sources of help or substances I recommend pay me anything. I have to keep this kind of integrity to keep your faith in me as a source of information.

Many people who have used my recommendations have recovered from their cancers. What percentage? Honestly, I don't know. I don't keep detailed records on these people. Nor do I follow up on them periodically to make sure they **maintain the lifestyle changes which got them well.** I know I have helped most of them get "cancer-free."

It is important for you to try to pin down the **cause** of your cancer. Then, I will explain to you exactly "what I would do if I were you" to reverse it. That is all I can offer you. It has been enough to heal thousands of people all over the world.

"What About My Doctor?"

A sensible question at this point is **"Don't I need a doctor?"** Certainly. We all need a doctor. If we need to be admitted to a hospital because of some trauma or other emergency illness, **we need a doctor.** I have a "family medicine" doctor who would perform that service for me. The question you will need to answer after you get your 20 hours or so of reading done is "Do I need a cancer doctor?"

My personal answer to that is **"No."** Not after he/she has used their diagnostic tools to confirm that I have cancer.

Later in this chapter, you will find several internet directories of **"holistic"** physicians. Most of these directories allow you to enter your Zip Code and find the ones closest to you. The doctor you choose to help you with your recovery from cancer is **a very personal decision.** He or she certainly **does not** have to be a cancer specialist (oncologist). I encourage you to search out that "perfect" physician. They are out there.

As you will see, however, you should not wait to begin your recovery regimen. You should start on that **now.** Use the guidance in Chapter 5 of this book and the other resources I will give you to begin **reversing the condition** which caused the cancer.

. Don't Fire Your Doctor -- Yet

As an informed consumer of medical service, you will be **empowered**. When the doctor's advice tracks with your knowledge, you'll **confidently accept** his/her treatment. When you need to, you will intelligently opt to **seek a second, third or fourth opinion**.

Unless your doctor is constantly studying microbiology, neurology, endocrinology, nutrition, immunology, alternative medicine and lots more disciplines, he/she is **not fully qualified** to advise you on beating your cancer. No human being can read and evaluate all the information currently available.

Put yourself in your doctor's shoes. She was trained in a medical school environment where **drug companies** provide most of the **research grants** and curriculum materials. Conventional (allopathic) medicine is taught to consist of treating "disease" and **symptoms** with **synthetic drugs and surgery**.

Once she is in practice, several drug company "representatives" every day **bombard** her, each leaving her free samples. A

Health Maintenance Organization (HMO) is looking over her shoulder, **criticizing** every diagnosis, every test. **Attorneys** await her least slip or recommendation of "unusual" treatment, misdiagnosis or prescription of the wrong drug. She is more and more **narrowly specialized**. Even keeping up with the information on studies in her own specialty is virtually impossible because of the demands of patient care on her time. Almost all of the new information she gets comes from "continuing education" sessions **sponsored by a drug company**.

With insurance companies and Medicare/Medicaid paying **only a fraction** of what she bills, she is under **extreme economic pressure** to keep patient "face-to-face" time to the bare minimum. One study showed that the average patient spends **only two minutes** with the doctor during each visit.

Is it any wonder that 51% of doctors in a recent large survey said they **would not go into medicine again** and 65% said they would **not recommend it to their children** as a career?

Even if they weren't so busy, there are very few doctors who **understand** the relations between lifestyle, environment and disease. The average M.D. received **two hours** (clock hours, not credit hours) on **nutrition and preventive medicine** in his six to ten years in medical school and hospital internship. Nutrition is a science **at least as complex** as conventional medicine.

You are fortunate that **thousands** of medical professionals have broken out of this "treat symptoms with drugs and procedures" mold. Soon, I will show you how to find one of these wonderful people near you.

I'm not offering medical advice. I'm not qualified to do that. Nothing you read here should be accepted as **medical opinion**.

However, I think I am qualified to offer you **information you may be unaware of** -- information which will help you locate a better medical professional and cooperate better with that doctor to **heal** your or your loved one's cancer.

Four Essentials

I have watched thousands of people battle cancer in the last seventeen years. Those who have been successful share four essentials. I call them the "4 A's." Memorize these and use them as a checklist frequently.

Essential #1: Attitude

Cancer is survivable. It doesn't matter what "stage" or type of cancer. All cancer patients can overcome it and live out their normal lifespan. People who believe this with all their heart and soul **get well**. Those who doubt it **don't**. It's that simple. Really.

Two things seem to characterize the cancer patients I've seen get well: First, they have decided to **take charge of their own health care**; and second, they have **committed 100%** to some regimen of diet and supplements.

How do you get and keep this commitment and positive attitude? **Gain knowledge** about the wide variety of cancer survivors and how they survived. Seek them out and talk to them. This is **not** a search for the **"magic bullet"** that heals all cancers. There is no such thing.

There are, however, literally **hundreds** of substances that are non-toxic and natural. Each one alone, or combined with others, has helped **thousands** of cancer patients get cancer-free. There are **simple life style changes** (diet, supplements, exercise, sunshine and emotional peace) that restore health to cancer patients. Many of them are quite **inexpensive** or even free.

Taking Charge of Your Own Health Care

You will not get this type of advice from your cancer doctor. You will usually be **urged** to begin chemotherapy and/or radiation immediately. For your best chance of recovery, **you must be prepared to resist this.** You, after all, **are in charge.** You should delay any decisions about interventions (surgery, chemo, radiation, etc.) until you are well enough informed to make an intelligent decision.

Believe the above paragraph and I can help you get well. Doubt it and I probably can't. Your training from childhood that **doctors have the answers** may make it hard for you to accept this. It takes **courage**.

While I have been able to help thousands of people around the world overcome their cancer, several friends and family members have succumbed to cancer during this same ten years. There is a saying that **"There is no prophet in his own home town."** When people I am close to do not follow my advice, it is painful and difficult for me to accept. However, the joy of hearing from one cancer survivor who has profited from my information inspires me to continue.

Keep an open mind. **Accept controversy** as a normal part of any treatment plan. Be strong. Family and friends are **well meaning**, but after a few hours of the research you have now started, they will know far less than you about cancer.

Essential #2: Advocate

If you have been diagnosed with cancer, you need to find your closest friend or relative and ask them to **be your advocate**. Cancer evokes emotions in almost everyone that are **hard to deal with**. Fear may freeze you. You are quickly exposed to confusing terms and **advice of all types** from well-meaning sources.

By reading this book, you are preparing yourself to **do battle** with the cancer "system." This battle is sometimes **difficult and stressful.** The path you are choosing is controversial. You need help and "moral" support.

You are going to need to do **research** to find the information and resources (doctors, clinics, supplements, etc.) you need. This research **does not** require a **great deal of time**, using this book as a guide to the information available on the Internet. We're talking about the equivalent of **1 or 2 ten-hour days** to become "smarter than your oncologist." Most cancer patients do not have either the **energy or patience** to devote this much time to getting "up to speed."

Your advocate needs to accompany you to **every** doctor's appointment. He or she must be committed to your recovery and have a **good sense of humor**. He or she must be willing to **discuss options with your doctor** and help you choose a second, third or fourth opinion doctor, if necessary.

A Quick Intro

If you don't believe my estimate of the time needed to "get smart," take a **half hour right now** and study this web site. Don't spend more than 30 minutes or so there right now. There is lots of useful information there. It is a non-commercial site – i. e. it is

not selling anything, just giving you information. For now, get a quick look at Webster Kehr's web site:
http://cancertutor.com ← must read

In summary, when your friend or loved one who is a cancer patient asks you to be their advocate, **accept gratefully**. There is no more spiritually fulfilling and uplifting role in this world. Your service will quite possibly **save your relative or loved one's life**. It most certainly will help him or her **avoid the drastic damage** done to their lifestyle and well being by the cancer "system."

Essential #3: Assistance (The Right Medical Professional)

This book will feature knowledge from **many M.D.s** and other medical professionals. All of them have broken the mold of the doctor who is concerned only with **treating symptoms** and **managing disease**. They have done unique research resulting in **breakthrough knowledge** about understanding the **causes** of cancer and treatments that work to **reverse it at the cellular level.** They are also concerned about prevention.

To help you understand what I mean, I will give you two examples.

First, **Dr. Matthias Rath** is a German M.D. who has gained worldwide recognition for his unique documentation of the **cause of cancer metastasis** (spreading of cancer cells to other parts of the body). He discovered and published this in the mid-1980's jointly with Linus Pauling, Ph.D., the famous physicist and winner of two Nobel prizes. Products based on their research are now readily available and are effective in **preventing metastasis,** the cause of 90% of cancer deaths.

8

Dr. Rath treats cancer of all types and stages (as well as heart disease and AIDS) using **Vitamin C** and two specific amino acids **(L-lysine and L-proline)**. He and his research VP travel all over the United States and Europe giving seminars on this subject (and, yes, selling his supplements at exorbitant prices). I have discovered a much cheaper source, which I will tell you about in Chapter 5. For Dr. Rath's explanation of the action of this compound, take a look at:

http://www.drrathresearch.org/sci_discoveries/cancer.html

For a second example, listen to Harold W. Harper, M.D. in a quote from his book *"How You Can Beat The Killer Diseases:"*

"What if cancer is a systemic, chronic, metabolic disease of which lumps and bumps constitute only symptoms? Will this not mean that billions of dollars have been misspent and that the basic premises on which cancer treatment and research are grounded are wrong? Of course it will, and in decades to come a perplexed future generation will look back in amazement on how current medicine approached cancer with the cobalt machine, the surgical knife, and the introduction of poisons into the system and wonder if such brutality really occurred."

How Do YOU Find One?

You would not have read this far unless you were interested in the help available from **alternative, complementary or integrative** medicine. So, how do you find a competent medical professional sympathetic to this approach to help you by supervising your recovery in your area? Fortunately, it is **not difficult** any more. Even folks in remote areas can usually find someone within 100 miles or so of their home. I have done it personally and helped many others, so I know exactly what is involved.

My Personal Experience

About five years ago, I decided to "walk the walk." I had been recommending to hundreds of cancer patients for two years that they find a qualified medical professional sympathetic to **Complementary & Alternative Medicine (CAM)**. I decided to find one that I could put my trust in for myself.

I called a unique "biological" dentist in San Antonio (where I lived at the time) who had treated my wife for her problems with root canals. I asked his wife, whom we had gotten to know because she worked in his office, **"Who would you go to in San Antonio if you were looking for a 'holistic healer?'"** She gave me four names. Two were osteopaths, one a naturopath and one a nutritionist. A friend of ours, who is also a nutritionist, had recommended **one of the same osteopaths** when I asked her the same question.

I interviewed all four of them -- three by telephone and e-mail and one in person. Among the questions I asked them were:

"If I should get prostate cancer, would you treat it?" Substitute your type of cancer. The answer you want is "Yes."

"I take a lot of supplements. How do you feel about that?" The answer you want is **"That is fine,"** not "Don't waste your money. Just eat a balanced diet."

"I feel you should help me, but that **I am in charge of my own health care**. Is that consistent with your approach?" The answer you want is, of course, an **enthusiastic** "Yes."

"How long have you been in practice?" Listen closely for the type of experience he/she has. Try to go into detail about previous practice sites, etc. in your interview. The value of his/her experience is strictly a **judgment call** on your part.

"Would you be willing to give me the **names of three of your patients** who would be willing to talk to me?" The answer you want is something like "If they agree after I call them, I'll be happy to give you their names."

The one I interviewed in person, as you might have guessed, was the osteopath recommended by both friends. He accepts Medicare. The others did not. He **did not charge** me for this initial interview, which lasted 40 minutes. He gave me all the right answers and we found we had a lot in common (military service, belief in alternative medicine, etc.). It was the first time in my life that I had spent that long talking to **any** medical professional about health matters.

I designated him as my Primary Care Physician. He treats cancer, along with all other medical problems, using both alternative and conventional means. In fact, he says he **"treats people, not disease."**

Your quest may not be as easy or rewarding as mine. But start with your **personal network** of friends and people in the medical profession – nurses, doctors, dentists, nutritionists, owners of health food stores, etc. Once you have exhausted that resource, go to one of the following websites and **search for people in your area.** It won't take you very long.

Using The Internet

Keep in mind, some alternative therapists may **not be allowed to treat cancer** depending upon the laws and politics of their country, region, state, province, etc. Don't let that discourage you. You can recover completely from cancer without the use of a medical professional. I know hundreds of people who have.

Here are some website directories of what I call "holistic" physicians. These may help you find the one you can trust. This is a **very personal decision** that nobody can make for you.

www.acam.org. The American College for Advancement In Medicine. This fine organization deserves special attention. Use their "Locate An ACAM Physician" link. You will find a searchable database of alternative practitioners and a toll-free number to call for assistance. Call the ones near you and discuss your situation. They may know other therapists near you offering a specific treatment you may want -- detoxification, for example.

www.lef.org/doctors.html. Here is a list of progressive doctors in all States in the U.S. and many other countries compiled by the Life Extension Foundation (LEF). As in the ACAM site above, these are generally open-minded individuals who understand and believe in alternative therapies.

www.naturopathic.org This is the website of the American Association of Naturopathic Physicians. It has a database searchable by zip code. This rapidly growing health care discipline seeks to discover the underlying cause of a disease and treat that rather than just eliminate symptoms, the approach used by the conventional medical establishment. Some states today, specifically Alaska, Arizona, Connecticut, Hawaii, Maine, Montana, New Hampshire, Oregon, Utah, Vermont, and Washington, license Naturopathic Doctors on a par with MDs.

www.cancure.org/home.htm An excellent site with many alternative doctors, hospitals and clinics from around the world. Put this website on your "favorites" list and come back to it to explore its cornucopia of information.

www.geocities.com/ray_m_89119/clinics.html Many links to alternative health websites, including many clinics in the U.S., Mexico and Germany.

http://nationalcenterforhomeopathy.org/resources/practitioners.js p At this site you will find some good guidance on selection of a homeopathic physician and a searchable database listing naturopaths, MDs, and other practitioners who use homeopathy. Homeopathy has been very popular in Europe for decades. England's Queen Elizabeth uses a homeopathic doctor.

www.holisticmedicine.org American Holistic Medical Association. Use the "Find A Doctor" button to explore their database of members of this organization.

www.nfam.org National Foundation for Alternative Medicine. This is an organization dedicated to information on the best alternative treatment information. A former American congressman named Berkley Bedell, who was cured of both lyme disease and prostate cancer by alternative means after his conventional doctors gave up on him, started it. Look under the "Resources" link for information.

www.whale.to/cancer/doctors.html. A list of doctors and clinics worldwide that may give you some leads.

Above all, **don't give up**. The truth is that there is a medical professional that will treat you and respect your wishes. All you have to do is find him or her.

Essential #4 – Action

Now for Essential #4. You **must start** treating yourself. Don't wait until you find the perfect medical professional. While you're searching for him or her, start taking supplements that are inexpensive, help **any** cancer and make it easier for you to regain your health (see Chapter 5). **Change your diet** using the guidelines in Chapter 5. Time is more important to you now than at any time in your life. Untreated cancer does not stop spreading. You must begin your battle **NOW.**

My recommended regimen usually **reverses cancer in 5 to 6 weeks.** If you can just avoid the conventional "therapy" – surgery, radiation and chemotherapy – for that long, you will probably be "cancer-free." These next few weeks are **critical** to your recovery. If you make intelligent and informed choices now, you can join the many people who have avoided the "cancer conveyer belt" of allopathic (conventional) medicine.

In summary, you need to keep in mind the four "A's."

- ➤ A Positive **Attitude**

- ➤ An **Advocate**

- ➤ **Assistance** (from A Competent Medical Professional)

- ➤ **Action** (Get Truckin')

In Chapters 5 and 7, I will discuss many of the available gentle, non-toxic cancer treatments in some detail. For now, I would like to help you understand two essentials for you to win your battle: 1) The cancer "environment" you are in; and 2) The true cause of cancer.

CHAPTER 2
THE CANCER ENVIRONMENT

"Most people would rather die than think. In fact they do."
Ralph Waldo Emerson

"Unproven Remedies"

In the past 70 years, hundreds of successful treatments for cancer have been discovered. You will find information on some of these in Chapters 5 and 7. Would it surprise you to know that **every one of these** is currently on the "Unproven Remedies" list maintained by the American Cancer Society (ACS)?

Doesn't it seem logical that **at least one** of these would have been thoroughly researched and investigated and found to have **some** use for at least **some** cancer sufferers? Isn't it mind-boggling that **every single one** is still labeled "unproven," in spite of the lapse of **decades** since their discovery?

But it's worse. Not only has our **cancer "system"** failed to prove and endorse these cures, the discoverers (most of them reputable M.D.s and researchers) have been **hounded** with lawsuits, license suspension and even jail sentences for treating cancer patients successfully. Many have been driven out of the country or into seclusion or even to suicide.

What do these treatments have in common? They are not approved by the Food and Drug Administration (FDA) for **treatment of any "disease"** and cannot be marketed as such. All contain **natural,** not synthetic, substances. Some have been patented, just like the pharmaceutical drugs. But they have not been through the "clinical" trial process, which, as we'll see, is largely bogus.

And yet, the U.S. alone has spent **thousands** of man-years and over **one hundred billion dollars** of government (your) money on cancer research just since the "War on Cancer" began in 1971. Cancer deaths per 100,000 people in the U.S., adjusted for age and population growth, are much higher today than in 1971.

Drug Company $$$$

You can only understand the cancer treatment "system" in the U.S. and, to a greater or lesser degree, in other countries, if you understand how much **power** the drug companies wield in our culture. Drugs used in cancer treatment are **all** produced and sold as **"chemotherapy."** What this means is that synthetic drugs must be compounded, and run through years (typically about **10 years**) of testing. This process costs between **$200 million and $500 million**.

Gene therapy and immune system vaccines have been researched for many years. They too must be tested through this **enormously expensive** system. There are lots of **natural immune system boosters** that are effective in fighting cancer. U.S. law prohibits them from being advertised as treatment for cancer or any other "disease."

Why not let "natural" remedies **co-exist** so people can make their own choices? That would seem logical, but there are Federal and State laws in the United States and other countries that **prohibit** this. Currently, under U. S. Federal law, **no natural substance** can be advertised as a cure for **any** condition – period. Companies that get too successful with cancer treatment are shut down by FDA lawsuits, supported *sub rosa* by the pharmaceutical companies. This is the environment you must learn to survive in (or **in spite of!**).

An Abominable Example

On July 12th, 2004, Lane Labs (the U.S. distributor for MGN-3, SkinAnswer, Shark Cartilage) was not only ordered to shut down, but to **reimburse all purchasers** of their products since 1999 by a Federal judge in New Jersey. Lane Labs, in the five years since the FDA began hounding them, had grown into a $30 million per year company. Their products had healed cancer of all types for **dozens** of my readers.

Drug Cartel Takes Over Europe

On March 13th 2002 the European Parliament – a 626-member legislature representing the 15 European Union countries – passed the "**EU Directive on Dietary Supplements.**" This is based on a United Nations Commission called "Codex Alimentarius Commission," formed in 1963.

This UN Commission had the innocuous goal of standardizing food production standards in all UN countries. In 1995, **Big Pharma** succeeded in getting the umbrella of this Commission expanded by the UN to cover food supplements. Now, with several drug company executives **in influential positions** in the EU Parliament, they have essentially **"passed a law against prevention."**

One German doctor, Dr. Matthias Rath (see above), claims to have collected 604 million signatures on a petition to block this "Directive." It passed anyway.

The effect is to make **300 food supplements** -- including chromium picolinate, yeast, lysine, selenium and even stevia (an herbal sweetener) – **illegal for over-the-counter sale**. Other supplements that remain in stores contain very low dosages. For example, the highest dose of Vitamin C available without a prescription is **100 mg**. For me to take my 3 grams a day, I'd have to take **30 tablets** instead of the three I take now.

Is It Coming To The U.S.?

There are rumors that the FDA is attempting to implement the **same restrictions in the U.S.** This despite the Dietary Supplement and Health Education Act (DSHEA) passed by Congress in 1994 to head off the last attempted power grab of this nature by the FDA. The DSHEA classifies supplements as food and allows manufacturers to inform the public about how supplements affect the "structure and function" of the body. The FDA, of course, has put many **restrictions** on this in the ensuing years. In fact, Lane Labs (see above) felt they were following the provisions of this law to the letter. Obviously, they got way too successful and **Big Pharma** pressured the FDA to shut them down.

Drug Marketing

The marketing of toxic drugs lies at the heart of the "war on cancer." For example, in one study, the **cost of drugs** was 55 percent of total treatment cost for small-cell lung cancer.

An article in the Journal of the American Medical Association (JAMA) recently stated that **oncologists** (cancer doctors) make an average of **$253,000 a year**, of which **75% is profit from chemotherapy drugs** administered in their offices.

If you have any doubts about the drug company omnipresence in our lives, all you have to do these days is **turn on your TV**. It seems like every other commercial is for some prescription drug. What's going on here?

In 1997, it became legal in the U.S. **for the first time** for drug companies to plug their wares **directly to the consumer** (you and me). In the years since then, the spending on TV and print advertising by Big Pharma in the U.S. has ballooned. This same type of advertising is still illegal in European countries, Australia and New Zealand.

Would you believe that in 2001 alone, the drug companies spent **$15.7 billion** (with a "b") on **TV and print ads for prescription drugs?** This is more than any other industry spends on advertising. More than the auto industry, the housing industry, retail giants like WalMart and so on.

Why? Well, it's pretty obvious. The **brainwashing** of the U.S. public continues. Got a problem? A prescription from your doctor is all you need to fix it. No need to worry about all those goody-two-shoes urging you to eat sensibly and exercise. Just jot down the latest name for a drug that just cost one of the international drug companies (Bristol-Myers-Squibb, Merck, etc.) $500 million to bring to market and go **bug your doctor** to write you a prescription for it. 12% of the prescriptions written in the U.S. happen just this way.

Just as important as the hype it gives their products is the **incredible clout** this spending gives the drug companies with the media. Why else would the media conveniently **fail to note** the unpleasant or **even lethal** side effects of prescription pharmaceuticals? These side effects are the **fourth leading cause of death** in the United States – right behind cancer, heart disease and stroke.

The U.S. spent **1.8 TRILLION DOLLARS** for health care in 2005. You might think most of this money went for hospital care.

Wrong!

Americans have spent **more on prescription drugs** than hospital care for the last several years. About two-thirds of this is wasted on drugs that only **treat symptoms** and allow the person to deteriorate without addressing the **underlying cause** of his/her disease.

Insane Profits

Are the drug companies crazy to spend $500 million to develop a drug? **Crazy like a fox!** Here is just one example. **AstraZeneca** is a drug company you have probably never heard of. According to Forbes magazine (March 18, 2002), they are the world's fourth-largest pharmaceutical company.

IN 2001 ALONE, AstraZeneca made **$630 million** on the sale of **Nolvadex** (a.k.a. tamoxifen), a breast cancer drug. This drug has been on the market **since 1973**. They made **$728 million** on the sale of **Zoladex**, a prostate/breast cancer drug. It was **introduced in 1987**. They made another **$569 million** on **Casodex**, another prostate cancer drug introduced in 1995. Within two years, says Forbes, this company's sales of **cancer fighter drugs alone** will top **$2.5 billion** a year.

One company, Bristol-Myers-Squibb, spends more than **one billion dollars** per year on research and employs 4,000 scientists and support personnel. It holds patents on **more than a dozen drugs** approved by the FDA for the treatment of cancer; this accounts for **almost half** of the chemotherapy sales in the world.

Influence – Far And Wide

Bristol-Myers-Squibb also **creatively influences** cancer research. It gives out awards, lectures and grants of many kinds. It pays for updates to orthodox cancer textbooks, and **supports research** and **"data management"** of clinical studies on its patented agents. Other cancer drug companies do the same.

Memorial Sloan-Kettering Cancer Center (MSKCC) in New York City is at the forefront of cancer research and has been for **at least the last 30 years**. Drug companies, again with Bristol-Myers-Squibb leading the way, occupy a **very strong position** at Memorial Sloan-Kettering. At one time, in 1995, for example:

➢ James D. Robinson III, the **Chairman** of the MSKCC **Board of Overseers and Managers,** was a **director of Bristol-Myers Squibb**.

➢ Richard L. Gelb, **Vice-Chairman** of the MSKCC board, was **chairman of the board of Bristol-Myers Squibb**.

➢ Richard M. Furland, MSKCC **board member**, retired in 1994 as the **president of Bristol-Myers Squibb**. He has also been a director of the Pharmaceutical Manufacturers Association.

➢ Benno C. Schmidt, **Honorary co-chairman** of MSKCC, was the **founder and board member of Genetics Institute**, a Massachusetts-based company that manufactures drugs for the cancer marketplace. He was also a **director of Gilead Sciences (which makes cancer-related drugs); Matrix and Vertex Pharmaceuticals**. He received the Bristol-Myers Squibb

Award for distinguished service to cancer research in 1979.

➤ Paul A. Marks, M.D., the **President and CEO** of MSKCC, was a **director of Pfizer**, which manufactures cancer-related drugs. He was also on the board of National Health Labs and of Life Technologies.

FDA – The Federal Watchdog?

Well, what about the federal government bureaucracy responsible for protecting you and me from such greed-oriented businesses, the FDA. Sorry, folks. This agency is even more **corrupted by drug money** than the EU Parliament.

One study recently showed that **55% of FDA executives** go to work for pharmaceutical companies when they leave the FDA. 20% of the FDA employees who work on the drug approval process are **actually paid** by the drug companies. Would you think they would be completely objective? Hmmmm.

In May, 2001, the Los Angeles Times published an article by David Willman entitled **"New FDA Policy Resulted in Seven Deadly Drugs."** He described how easier FDA standards on drug approval were prescribed by Congress in 1993. After a two-year investigation, the L.A. Times reported that in "adverse event" reports filed with the FDA, the **seven drugs** were cited as suspects in **1,002 deaths**. Because the deaths are reported by doctors, hospitals and others on a **voluntary basis**, the true number of deaths **could be much higher**, according to epidemiologists.

The seven drugs – Lotronex, Rezulin, Posicor, Redux, Rotashield, Propulsid and Raxar – are among the **hundreds of**

new drugs approved by the FDA since 1993. A telling statistic: these seven drugs alone generated **$5 billion** in U.S. sales **before they were pulled from the market** by the FDA. Another interesting statistic: In 1988, **only 4%** of the new drugs introduced into the world market were approved first by the FDA. In 1998, the FDA's first-in-the-world approvals had **spiked to 66%!**

Once the world's safety leader, the FDA was the **last to withdraw** several new drugs in the late 1990s that were banned by health authorities in Europe.

Doctors Comment On The FDA

"This track record is totally unacceptable," said Dr. Curt Furberg, a professor of public health sciences at Wake Forest University. *"The patients are the ones paying the price. They're the ones developing **all the side effects**, fatal and non-fatal. Someone has to speak for them."*

It's not that doctors didn't speak up against these drugs. *"They've lost their compass and they forget who it is that they are ultimately serving,"* said **Dr. Lemuel Moye,** a University of Texas School of Public Health physician who served from 1995 to 1999 on an **FDA advisory committee**. *"Unfortunately, the public pays for this, because the public believes that the FDA is watching the door, that they are the sentry."*

The FDA's shift is felt directly in the private practice of medicine, said Dr. William Isley, a Kansas City, Missouri diabetes specialist. He implored the agency to **reassess Rezulin four years ago** after a patient he treated suffered **liver failure** taking the pill.

"FDA used to serve a purpose," Isley said. *"A doctor could feel sure that a drug he was prescribing was **as safe as possible**. Now you wonder what kind of evaluation has been done, and what's been **swept under the rug**."*

"The Truth About The Drug Companies"

In August 2004, Dr. Marcia Angell (an M.D.) published a very interesting book. It is entitled *"The Truth About The Drug Companies : How They Deceive Us and What To Do About It."* Dr. Angell's perspective is particularly interesting because for 20 years before her retirement in 2000, she was **executive editor and editor-in-chief of the New England Journal of Medicine,** one of the most prestigious medical journals in the world. Under her watch, the journal published **hundreds of studies** of new drugs. It also published blunt editorials harshly critical of the pharmaceutical industry and the way drugs are tested and approved in the United States. She makes several major points, in an interview published in the Los Angeles Times, which are critical for you to understand:

> ➤ *"Drugs are expensive, but not because of the costs of research. The money the largest drug companies spend on marketing and the amount of profit they make dwarfs their research expenditures. In 2002, for example, the biggest drug companies spent only about 14% of sales on research and development and 31% on what most of them call 'marketing and administration.' They consistently make more in profits than they spend on R & D. And their profits are immense. In 2002, the combined profits of the 10 drug companies in the Fortune 500 were $35.9 billion. That's more than the profits of the other 490 businesses put together, if you subtract losses from gains."*

➢ *"…the number of truly innovative new drugs is quite small. True, many drugs are coming to market. But most of them aren't new at all. They are minor variations of best-selling drugs that are already on the market."*

➢ *"Drug makers are only required to show that a new medication is more effective than a placebo, or sugar pill. If a drug works better than a placebo and is safe, the FDA approves it, and it can enter the market. The result is that doctors don't know if a new drug that comes along is any better or worse than the drugs they're already using."*

➢ *"…patents run out on older drugs and they can then be sold as generics at as little as 20% of the price (they sold at while still under patent). Pharmaceutical manufacturers need a constant supply of new drugs that have patent protection so they can charge whatever they want."*

➢ *"…why are drug companies spending so much on marketing? The answer is that they have to convince us that their me-too drugs are better than the others. And that takes a heap of marketing, because there's usually no scientific evidence to back up the claim."*

The FDA Responds

The FDA's response: *"All drugs have risks; **most of them have serious risks**,"* said Dr. Janet Woodcock, director of the FDA's drug-review center. *"Once a drug is proven effective and safe"* [in the case of chemotherapy drugs, half the test subjects survive it!], Woodcock says, *"the FDA depends on doctors to take into account the risks, **to read the label**…We have to rely on the* *practitioner community to be the **learned intermediary**. That's why drugs are prescription drugs."*

Dr. Woodcock alluded in a recent interview to the difficulty she feels in rejecting a proposed drug that might have cost a company **$150 million or more** to develop.

The "Bottom Line"

Dr. Woodcock, how many people have you heard of who have been killed by an overdose of Vitamin C or by eating too many vegetables?

Question All Medications

Do you see how important it is to "second guess" your doctor? **Question everything.** If you or your loved one are being prescribed a medication [especially chemotherapy], **ALWAYS** ask to see the statistical studies and warning labels which are **required to be read by physicians**. Obviously, they don't have the time to study them all. You **MUST take the time**. Your life or your loved one's life may be in danger.

Suppression of Competition

The logical question is "Why does the FDA and the EU go to such lengths to **suppress** non-toxic treatments for cancer and other diseases?" The only answer is that our medical system, in the U.S., Europe, Australia and other countries has become dominated by **drug company money**.

Conspiracy?

The true nature of the Big Pharma influence on governmental and private agencies can only be appreciated with **a lot more**

detail than I can provide you here. The best way to appreciate this problem I know of is to read a book called **"Politics in Healing – The suppression and manipulation of American Medicine" by Daniel Haley**. It was published in 2000 and is available from amazon.com.

After 10 years of research, Haley has documented **12 case studies** of systematic suppression of **proven cures – mostly for cancer**. Substances like Glyoxilide, Krebiozen, DMSO, Colustrum, Hydrazine Sulfate, 714X, Aloe Vera and Cesium Chloride are covered in great detail along with names like Royal Rife, Harry Hoxsey, Dr. William Koch, Dr. Andrew Ivy, Gaston Naessens, Dr. Robert Becker and Dr. Stanislaw Burzynski.

Here's what Julian Whitaker, M.D., prominent leader in alternative medicine says about this book:

"Daniel Haley has written a very important book about the medical profession, detailing the struggles between good and evil as no one ever has before. Incredible as these stories are, they are true!"

The suppression Daniel Haley documents has been an **obvious conspiracy** among the American Medical Association (AMA), the American Cancer Society (ACS), the National Institutes of Health (NIH), the FDA and the Federal Trade Commission (FTC) to serve the **Big Pharma cartel**.

This is not an easy book to read. As I finished each chapter at night, I would grumble to my wife about the **evils of big money** corruption in our country and the millions of people dying needlessly because of it. Nevertheless, it should be **required reading** for everyone in the world.

If you are in a hurry to discover the best ways to treat your or your loved ones cancer, I will forgive you if you put off reading this book. However, when you get the time, please **come back to it**. You will never look on our medical or political systems the same way again. In the meantime, if you must press on, please take my word for the need for you to exercise **great caution** in accepting anything you hear from your "conventional" (or "allopathic") medicine system without confirmation from several sources outside that system.

Should We Blame The Doctors?

Is your doctor a part of this conspiracy? **No.** Most doctors are dedicated, over-worked, even **heroic** champions of the restoration of their patients' health. Unfortunately for you, they are **products of a medical system** that is closed to innovation in very important ways. Most do not even consider treatments that do not fit the mold they have been **taught in medical school** and in all "continuing education" since. In fact, most of the "continuing education" of doctors is done on junkets to exotic destinations **sponsored by the drug companies**.

What is the current **medical dogma** on cancer by which oncologists live? First, that cancer is a **foreign enemy** in the body that must be **attacked.** The only acceptable treatment is to cut it out, poison it or burn it. Second, that all **patented synthetic drugs** (chemotherapy, etc.) approved for them to prescribe are **superior to any natural, non-toxic substance** for cancer therapy. And finally, that food supplements are a **waste of money** for those who eat a "balanced diet." These three "wrong paradigms" almost insure that you will need to question their judgment.

Please don't just accept or reject my views on this. Check out some information from **real experts**. One example is the following article. The authors, Nicholas Regush, an experienced health reporter for ABC News and Dr. Joseph Mercola, one of the best-qualified medical professionals I have ever encountered, are certainly **not radical revolutionaries**. Their views are important to you, however, because you need to understand **what you are up against** in your use of our conventional medical system. Please read this article:

http://www.mercola.com/2002/feb/27/death_of_medicine.htm

The Cancer Industry

In his interesting book *World Without Cancer – The Story of Vitamin B17*, G. Edward Griffin puts it this way:

"With billions of dollars spent each year in research, with additional billions taken in from the cancer-related sale of drugs, and with vote-hungry politicians promising ever-increasing government programs, we find that, today, there are more people making a living from cancer than dying from it. If the riddle were to be solved by a simple vitamin, this gigantic commercial and political industry could be wiped out overnight. The result is that the <u>science</u> of cancer therapy is not nearly as complicated as the <u>politics</u> of cancer therapy."

Legislation claiming to protect the consumer of drugs is usually **written by** the drug industry. Politicians who are grateful for the financial support of the drug companies are eager to put their names on legislation and push for its enactment. Once it becomes law, it serves merely to **protect** the sponsoring drug companies against competition. Competition from natural cancer treatments, for example. The consumer is **the victim** of this legislation, not the beneficiary.

In drug testing and marketing, unlike other industries that lobby Congress, there is the added necessity to pretend that everything is being done scientifically. Therefore, in addition to recruiting the aid of politicians, **scientists** must also be enlisted – a feat that is easily accomplished by the judicious allocation of funding for research.

Some History

This process is nothing new. Former FDA Commissioner James L. Goddard, in a **1966** speech before the Pharmaceutical Manufacturers Association, expressed concern about **dishonesty in testing** new drugs. He said:

"I have been shocked at the materials that come in. In addition to the problem of quality, there is the problem of dishonesty in the investigational new drug usage. I will admit there are gray areas in the IND [Investigation of New Drug] situation, but the conscious withholding of unfavorable animal clinical data is not a gray area. The deliberate choice of clinical investigators known to be more concerned about industry friendships than in developing good data is not a gray area."

Goddard's successor at the FDA was Dr. Herbert Ley. In 1969, he testified before the Senate committee and described several cases of **blatant dishonesty** in drug testing. One case involved an assistant professor of medicine who had tested **24 drugs for 9 different companies**. Dr. Ley said:

"Patients who died while on clinical trials were not reported to the sponsor… Dead people were listed as subjects of testing. People reported as subjects of testing were not in the hospital at the time of the tests. Patient consent forms bore dates indicating they were signed after the subjects died."

Another case involved a **commercial drug-testing firm** that had worked on 82 drugs from 28 companies. Dr. Ley continued:

"Patients who died, left the hospital, or dropped out of the study were replaced by other patients in the tests without notification in the records. Forty-one patients reported as participating in studies were dead or not in the hospital during the studies… Record-keeping, supervision and observation of the patients in general were grossly inadequate."

Money corrupts. Really big money **corrupts completely**!!

The Lancet Nails Drug Company Research

For a view on this subject from an **impeccable source**, I suggest you read a recent article from *The Lancet*, the esteemed British medical journal. It covers research funded by drug companies and was posted by **Dr. Joseph Mercola** in his great newsletter. You can read the article and Dr. Mercola's comments on it at:

http://www.mercola.com/2002/nov/20/drug_companies.htm

While you are there, sign up for Dr. Mercola's newsletter. It is a treasure trove of health information delivered twice weekly to your e-mail box. It's free.

A Personal Anecdote

In 1996, my urologist prescribed **Hytrin**, a drug manufactured by **Abbott Laboratories**, for my enlarged prostate. It was quite effective in reducing my nocturnal ups and downs. It relaxes the prostate and bladder muscles. Hytrin is also used to treat high blood pressure, which I don't have.

For the first three and a half years, my co-payment for Hytrin was **$60**. I needed a refill about once a month. When I asked the pharmacist if there was a generic, he said no, that Abbott Labs had a **patent** on it and only the named drug could be sold.

Well, guess what? In the middle of 2000, I happily found that Abbott Labs patent had **expired**. I found out only because my pharmacist filled my prescription with the generic (terazosin hydrochloride) and my co-payment was **$5**, instead of $60.

The plot thickens. In September 2000, I received a letter from my urologist's office. They were running a **clinical trial** on a "new" drug to treat enlarged prostates and they wanted **volunteers** for the test. I was curious, so I called them. It turned out that this office, the **largest urology clinic in San Antonio**, had a specialized staff for drug testing.

They asked me a few questions. Apparently, I qualified and they asked me to participate in the test -- what's called a **Random Clinical Trial**. It requires the participants to take no medication (stop the terazosin) for one month and then try the "new" medication for three months -- unless, of course, you got the **placebo** (sugar pill), which neither you nor the docs would know about. One half of the people would get the "new" drug and **one half the placebo**.

Guess what the "new" drug was? Not hard, was it. It was **Hytrin II**. A "new", and, of course, **newly patented** form of the drug. It was supposed to "improve the quality of the treatment" of BPH (Benign Prostatic Hypertrophy), which is what I, and most males my age, have, an enlarged prostate gland. I politely declined to participate in the clinical trial.

What's **wrong** with this picture? Well, several things:

1) Do you think it is **coincidental** that Abbott Labs just finished developing Hytrin II **a few months** after their patent for Hytrin I ran out?

2) Do you think it is **ethical** for a large urology clinic to act as the agent for a drug manufacturer in a clinical trial? Isn't this something of a **conflict of interest**? The rumor is that they get $8,000 per recruit from the drug company.

3) Do you think either Abbott Labs or my doctor thought about the **financial impact** of a "new" drug on me or other seniors?

4) Why do you think the presidential race in 2000 made a BIG DEAL out of a **"prescription drug benefit"** for seniors? Why did Congress pass a law enacting this in 2003? Could it have something to do with the **political contributions** from the drug companies? Remember, that prescription drug benefit comes right out of **taxpayers' pockets**. And why didn't the bill setting up this new "benefit" entitle the federal government to negotiate drug prices, just like they do in the Veterans Administration drug program? Could the fact that Big Pharma has 1.430 full-time lobbyists in Washington, D.C. alone have anything to do with it?

5) Why aren't we debating about how to keep the drug companies from **gouging** Americans while they sell the same drug at **one-fifth the cost** in Europe and Canada?

Relief From Canada

In September 2000, William Raspberry, wrote a column in the Washington Post about *"One Long-Term Cure for High Drug Prices."* Here are a few paragraphs from that article:

"There are at least two pieces of the problem of high cost of prescription drugs, Rep. Bernie Sanders, an independent from Vermont, has been saying for some time now.

But most of the political and journalistic focus has been on only one piece: The 'outrageously high price' of medications. He'd like to call attention to the other half of the problem: The fact that Americans 'are paying by far the highest prices in the world for the same exact drug – not a generic, but the same exact drug.'

The solution, he says is simplicity itself. Allow registered pharmacies and drug distributors to purchase FDA-approved drugs anywhere in the world for resale here. Reimportation, he calls it in the bill he hopes will pass Congress before the campaign recess."

[NOTE: The bill passed and was signed into law by President Clinton. The Bureau of Health and Human Services never wrote regulations to implement it because they were concerned for the "safety" of consumers....Hmmmm]

"'This is important stuff,' Sanders said in a telephone interview from his Burlington office. 'I traveled to Canada with a group of women with breast cancer, and we looked at the price of tamoxifen, a drug that is widely prescribed for the treatment of breast cancer. You could get it in Canada for a 10th of the U.S. price.

If this bill were to go into effect tomorrow, U.S. pharmacies would be purchasing tamoxifen in Canada and retailing it here at 30 to 50 percent less than they now charge.'

Sanders says the same thing applies to any number of drugs – all approved by the FDA and originally manufactured in or exported from the United States.

'Pharmacies should be able to purchase these drugs the same way other companies purchase shoes, slacks or washing machines,' he says.

…The biggest obstacle to passage this term is the pharmaceutical industry, Sanders says. 'They are the most powerful lobbying force on Capitol Hill,' he said. 'They've spent tens of millions in opposition of this bill.'"

So What?

Where does all this leave you, the cancer patient or caregiver? Well, hopefully, it leaves you **somewhat skeptical** about claims by the cancer "industry" that all therapies not sold by Bristol-Myers-Squibb or Merck or Abbott Labs or whoever are **"unproven"** and therefore pure **"quackery."**

As a bare minimum, to avoid what happened to Marjorie, my former wife, and me, you **must** educate yourself. You must be prepared to get more than one opinion. Then, when you've found the doctor (or homeopath or naturopath) that you trust, you **must be prepared to co-doctor** with him or her throughout your treatment.

This book is designed to end your **blind** faith and trust in our system of cancer "therapy" and arm you with the power to search beyond it. Faith is fine, if it derives from the power of knowledge and trust in your physician.

You Have The Power -- Use It

I'm going to arm you with **information** -- from books, the Internet, newsletters, magazines and any other source. You will be able to **take charge** of your health. I am hoping you will not be satisfied with **treating symptoms**. You will want to **treat causes**.

But before you can treat causes, you need to understand them.

Seventeen years ago, one of my wife's cancer surgeons told me, *"80% of it is still mystery to us."* At the time, I didn't know what he meant. Now, I think I do.

What he meant was that what happens in your body **at the cellular level** is indeed mystery to almost all doctors.

➢ Interactions between your **brain** and your **immune system**.
➢ What emotional and other **stress** does to your immune system.
➢ How **your mouth** can affect the rest of your body.
➢ Exactly what **chemotherapy** does to your immune system.
➢ How the side effects of chemo can be **offset with natural substances**.
➢ What the **long term** effects of chemotherapy are.
➢ What other treatments are available to **recover from cancer**.
➢ How **non-toxic substances** can boost your immune system.

➢ What organs are affected by **nutritional** deficiencies (or excesses).
➢ How **cells react** to food and medicine.
➢ How exercise and nutrition affect diseases like **diabetes**.
➢ What **"free radicals"** do to your health.
➢ Which **antioxidants** are the most effective against free radicals.
➢ What **natural substances** provide your body with antioxidants.
➢ **...and many, many more.**

You MUST Be Careful?

You **must not trust** everything you are told by a person with M.D. after their name. You must **monitor** everything that is done to your loved one in a hospital. That means spending the night in their hospital room with him/her. I have found that it is very hard to convince many people of those **two simple facts**. If you have had that same frustrating experience, here are a few statistics that might help you next time.

Doctors are officially the third leading cause of death in the United States. In causing the death of their patients, they trail only cancer and heart disease. There are currently more than (probably **much** more than) 250,000 deaths per year from **iatrogenic** causes. That strange word means **"induced in a patient by a physician's words or actions."** Here's the published breakdown for 1999:

12,000 Unnecessary surgery
7,000 Medication errors in hospitals
20,000 Other errors in hospitals
80,000 Infections in hospitals
106,000 Non-error, negative effects of drugs

This information is from an article by Dr. Barbara Starfield of the John Hopkins School of Hygiene and Public Health in the *Journal of the American Medical Association* (JAMA Vol 284, July 26, 2000). The above statistics come from the review process that happens after every death in a hospital to determine the true cause of each death for insurance purposes and to get **smarter about treatment**.

Unfortunately, the hospitals seem to be **losing the latter battle**. If you think those numbers have gotten smaller in ensuing years, you're much more of an optimist than I am.

Do you really think hospitals accurately report that it was the chemotherapy **treatment** itself that **killed the patient**? A good estimate I've seen is that **at least 80%** of the 570,000 deaths each year attributed to "cancer" in the U.S. were actually **caused by the cancer "therapy."** Furthermore, when a cancer patient treated with chemotherapy or radiation dies from infections like pneumonia caused by the damage to their immune system, their death is not a "cancer death."

In Canada, where they have "socialized" medicine, it seems that doctors can be somewhat more frank than they can in the U.S. The **McGill Cancer Center** in Montreal, Quebec, one of the largest and most prestigious cancer treatment centers in the world, did a study of oncologists to determine how they would respond to a diagnosis of cancer. On the confidential questionnaire, 58 out of 64 oncologists (91%) said that **ALL chemotherapy programs were unacceptable to them and their family members.** The overriding reasons they gave for this decision were that the drugs are **ineffective** and have an **unacceptable degree of toxicity**. These are the same doctors who will tell you that their chemotherapy treatments will shrink your tumor and prolong your life!

A similar and more recent study conducted by the Los Angeles Times found that **75%** of the oncologists stated that chemotherapy and radiation were **unacceptable as treatments for themselves or their families**. Yet, as of today, 75% of cancer patients take chemotherapy. Go figure!

Are you sufficiently skeptical about medical advice? Good! Let's get down to the business of making you "smarter than your oncologist." Let's first take a look at what cancer is and what causes it.

CHAPTER 3
WHAT IS CANCER?

*"The Philosophies of one age have become the Absurdities of
the next and the Foolishness of yesterday has become the
Wisdom of tomorrow."*
Sir William Osler (1902)

Cancer is Simply...

A cancer diagnosis scares **all of us**. I have **no more vivid
memory** than seeing my former wife's body after it had been
wracked by **four years of cancer**, chemotherapy, operations
and painkilling drugs.

Her bout with cancer started me on my search for answers. How
can we deal with it **gently**? How can we **prevent** it? To do either,
we must first **understand** it.

Some Cancer Numbers

First, let me give you a few numbers. As of 2004, cancer is the
leading cause of death in the United States. About 24% of all
deaths each year are blamed on cancer.

Notice the word "about". As I mentioned above, my former wife,
Marjorie, died on November 1, 1994 after a **four-year bout** with
cancer. On her death certificate, her doctor wrote **"heart failure"**
as the cause of death. Obviously, any statistics on death rates
need to be taken with a grain of salt. My doctor friends tell me
that the law requires them to enter the **final** cause of death, not
the **precursor,** whatever that means.

More than a **million** Americans are diagnosed with cancer **each year** and more than half a million death certificates cite cancer as the cause of death.

Another 800,000 develop **small, "non-invading" cancers** and various mild kinds of skin cancer. Both types generally do not spread and can be easily removed. These cancers are **not counted** in the annual cancer statistics.

For **women 35 to 74**, cancer is the leading cause of death. For **men** of the same age range, cancer is **second** only to cardiovascular disease as the leading cause of death.

Despite the high incidence of cancer and our federal government's **"War on Cancer",** begun in 1971 and supported by over $100 billion dollars of research, virtually **no progress** has been made in healing the most common forms of cancer.

According to the World Health Organization, there were **10 million new cases** of cancer in 1996, and in 2001 they predicted a yearly total of **14.7 million**. These numbers have continued to grow. They are so huge that the suffering they imply is incomprehensible.

In the United States, the death rate from cancer had **risen 8%** by 2004 from 1970, just before the "War on Cancer" was launched. Despite the large number of people who have **stopped smoking** in recent years, according to the National Cancer Institute, the incidences for some of the most common cancers -- colon, breast, prostate, etc. -- are **sharply increasing.**

To put it another way, **every other man** and **every third woman** in the United States will get cancer -- unless we understand it better and make the lifestyle changes I will show you.

If a tumor is found early and removed, it will not **regrow or appear elsewhere about 50%** of the time. Once a cancer has **metastasized** (spread to other sites in the body), chemotherapy and/or radiation will heal it permanently only about **3% of the time**. I don't like those odds and would not accept them. Will you?

Where Does It Come From?

Most cancers arise from our interaction with the world around us. Almost **one-third** of all cancers diagnosed in Europe and in the United States can be linked to **tobacco** use. These account for more than 150,000 deaths in the United States each year.

Food choices contribute to another one-third of the cancers, especially stomach and colon cancers.

Thinner people are at **lower risk** of breast, prostate and uterine cancer. This is probably because these cancers are linked to high exposure to the sex hormones, estrogen and testosterone. These hormones are **stored in fat**.

People who drink **alcohol** excessively have higher levels of **mouth and liver** cancer.

Occupational hazards, such as **asbestos and formaldehyde**, account for about **5%** of all cancers.

Surprisingly, only about 3% of cancers are due to hereditary factors. Where clusters of cancers occur in a family, the cause is almost always similar **lifestyle choices** – particularly diet.

Probably the most important thing to know about the cause of cancer is that in most cases it occurs as a result of: 1) an **emotional trauma** such as loss of a child in a dramatic way or

extended emotional stress like that caused by a bitter divorce; or 2) **root canal teeth**. Both of these suppress the immune system and allow cancer (an opportunistic condition) to grow; and 3) **what we put in our mouth** – sure, cigarettes and alcohol, but also our food. Cooked food has no enzymes and few nutrients. The lack of nutrients and the huge number of chemicals in all supermarket food is a major scandal and responsible for millions of deaths each year.

What Exactly Is Cancer?

Cancer means the **growth of tumors**. It's a category that includes a broad range of (what your doctor calls) **"diseases."** These include lymph system cancers called "lymphoma," blood borne cancers like "leukemia," and skin cancers such as "melanoma." Obviously, not all cancers involve tumors.

As you will see, I do not believe cancer, or any other degenerative condition, is a "disease." More accurately, it is a **"reaction."** Usually, it is a reaction to the lifestyle choices you have made over the last several years. Where emotional trauma or root canal teeth are not involved, the cause is almost always diet.

About 3 to 4% of all cancers stem from inherited genes. The other 96 to 97% are caused by a breakdown in cellular communication. Attempts to explain the cause of this breakdown **vary widely**. Some say that **"microbes"** inside the cells create the cancer cells; others say **"free radicals"** damage the DNA; others say a coating of **indigestible proteins** on the cell membrane; others say a drop in the cell's **"voltage;"** others say **acidity**. As you can see, the exact cause is not agreed upon by all experts.

One thing is certain: If your body (particularly your immune system) is **healthy enough** to fight off all the toxins it takes in or which reside in it, you don't get the "reaction" called cancer.

One thing common to all cancers is **damage to the DNA** in the cell nucleus. This DNA is **duplicated with every cell division**. Average adults have 75 trillion cells in their body. Once again – **75,000,000,000,000 cells**. 99% of the cells in our bodies are called "somatic" cells. All of our cells except brain and nerve cells get replaced thousands or hundreds of thousands of times during our lifetime. In **seven years** this process of cell division and death replaces virtually **every cell** in our bodies.

Another way to look at this is that **every day** about **29 billion cells** get replaced in our body. Why is this important? Because inevitably "mistakes" occur during this process, probably from one of the "causes" mentioned above. If these mistakes in the cell's DNA occur only .003% (three thousandths of a percent) of the time, we produce a **million cancer cells** every day. This is probably conservative. A billion (with a "b") cancer cells are about the size of the eraser on a pencil.

Division Problems

When a cell divides, the DNA in that cell is copied and passed on to the new cell. But the DNA in any one cell can become damaged. Pieces of the instructions on the genes can get **knocked out or changed** – mutated.

If this mutation occurs in the wrong place – in an active gene, for instance – it can **disrupt the function of the cell**, causing it to lose its ability to survive with normal "respiration." Yes, each cell breathes in oxygen and breathes out energy.

Your beautiful body includes a **regulatory system** that is mind-boggling. For example, when you get a simple cut on your hand, your cells go to work to repair the damage. When enough cells have gathered around the cut to heal it, the cells **stop dividing**. Ever wonder why? Because there is a **"suicide gene"** in the DNA which says "Enough, already."

Not only is the total number of cells kept in check, but also **"proofreader"** genes in the DNA look for abnormalities in the cell. When they find one, they either fix it or kill the cell. They are on duty 24/7. Isn't this stuff **amazing**?

Your **immune system** (about 20 trillion of the 75 trillion cells) also kills off these damaged cells by the millions every day. It is your **second line of defense** against abnormal cells.

So, cancerous (dividing out of control) cells occur in our body **every day**. If the cell's own "policing" mechanisms fail, the immune system needs to **recognize this "wayward" cell and kill it**. But, the immune system is nothing but **specialized cells**. The immune system's 130 different types of cells live in the same "environment" as the rest of our body's cells. What if they are weakened by the same process that caused the dividing cell's "abnormality" – what then?

The cell has **lost its "suicide"** function. The **"proofreader"** gene missed the mistake. Your immune system **is too weak** to provide its normal second line of defense. Result: **The Big C.**

The cancer cells usually travel to the **weakest and most acid organ** in your body and you have a tumor. The cancer tumor grows because the **"daughter"** cells inherit the same abnormal genes. When it is finally diagnosed, the cancer tumor has often been growing for 5-15 years.

The Cancer Tumor

Let's take a look at a typical cancer tumor. Let's say it is in the colon, for example. A tumor (a symptom of cancer) is some number (usually billions) of cancer cells surrounded by tissue. Cancer cells cannot grow tissue. In fact, they are relatively "dumb" cells. The cancer tumor is our body's **"emergency response"** to abnormal cells which are out of control. Our body tries to "wall them off" from the rest of its cells to limit the damage.

Of course, the cancer cells continue to divide out of control and the tumor grows. At some point, the effect of the tumor is "recognized" by you or your doctor. You feel a lump or you experience abnormal bleeding or pain, for example. Typically, at that point, your cancer doctor will perform some sort of exploratory **"procedure."** Usually, this is a "biopsy." A biopsy is literally **poking a hole** in the tumor tissue to remove a sample of the cells inside the tumor for testing in the lab.

How healthy do you think this is? Well, you're right. It is **not healthy**. Breaking the integrity of the tissue around the tumor frequently results in the spread of the cancer cells. Without this "procedure," they might have otherwise remained "contained" **inside the tumor tissue.**

Removal of the tumor using surgery always has the **same effect**. The surgeon says **"We got it all,"** when, in fact, he/she got **most** of the cancer cells and some escaped this "procedure." So, is it always smart to refuse biopsies and surgery? Biopsies, yes. Surgery, no. There are rare instances where surgery or "gamma knife" procedures to **"debulk"** the tumor are necessary – some brain tumors and colon tumors, for example.

You want to know what I would do? Simply avoid any "procedure" which might cause the spread (metastasis) of the cancer cells unless my life was immediately at stake. I know that a tumor will rarely kill me, whether it is malignant (growing) or not. With a regimen (see Chapter 5) which will bring **almost all cancers under control within six weeks**, there is rarely a need for invasive "procedures."

What Are Free Radicals?

Free radicals, one of the most common causes of cancerous DNA damage, **are** under your control. What are free radicals? Every day, we produce or take in millions of them. They are compounds that have **one unpaired electron** in their atomic makeup.

Try as you might, you **cannot avoid** free radicals. They are in your body and in the atmosphere. They result from the process your body uses to break down food, among **many other causes**. But they are also caused, and can be controlled, by the lifestyle decisions we make every day. What lifestyle decisions? Want a few examples?

- ➤ **Cigarette smoking** causes the largest number of free radicals of any lifestyle activity. Eventually, the number of free radicals it produces overcomes your body's elaborate defenses and you, the smoker, get lung cancer, emphysema, heart disease, and many more maladies.

- ➤ The **more "bad" fat** you take in, the **more free radicals** you produce. Particularly damaging are trans-fatty acids found in abundance in the "Standard American Diet" (SAD). McDonald's French fries, for example, have one of the highest concentrations of trans-fatty acids of any food.

➢ Food and vitamins and other supplements provide **"anti-oxidants"** which can kill off the free radicals by the **billions.**

➢ All of these lifestyle choices are **cumulative** – for better or worse.

In addition to cancer, free radical damage also causes senility, arthritis, hardening of the arteries, and the declining function of your immune system as you age.

Dietary Deficiencies

The **lack of nutrients** in our diet and what to do about it is the subject of many books. Several of the better ones are mentioned in Booklet #1 (at the end of this book) and Appendix A. **Leaching of the soil** by poor crop rotation along with **the way food is processed** ensure that our cells lack the nutrients they need to remain healthy. In fact, they are bombarded with hundreds of chemicals used in processed food every day.

Supplements and organic food can correct these problems to a certain extent. However, these conditions are the cause of **virtually all degenerative "reactions"** (arthritis, multiple sclerosis, diabetes, heart disease, fibromyalgia, chronic fatigue syndrome – and **certainly cancer** and many more).

Helping Your Immune System

A multitude of studies in recent years confirm the immune system's function in both preventing and **healing** cancer. Almost every day a new study is published in the search for drugs and vaccines that boost the immune system's ability to fight off cancer.

As we will see in Chapter 5, these drugs are **not necessary**. At least a dozen substances that are **non-toxic and harmless** to take have been proven to boost your immune system's ability to "mop up" abnormal cancerous cells.

Here's a quote from an interesting book, "Real Age", by Michael F. Roizen, M.D.:

*"As you age, your second line of defense, your immune system, tends to be less vigilant and does not as readily detect and destroy these abnormalities. The weaker your immune system, the more likely that it will not provide the necessary backup. The longer you live, the more likely that you will get improper cell divisions, the more likely that the DNA in a specific cell will contain a mutation, and the more likely that your immune system won't be there to catch a mistake. The most important thing to remember is this: **You can slow, and even reverse, the rate of aging of your immune system.**"* [Emphasis added].

Dr. Roizen goes on to explain causes and prevention measures for various types of cancer. If you would like to read more of his work, his book is called *REAL AGE --Are You as Young as You Can Be?* Copyright 1999 by Michael F. Roizen, M.D. Also, check out his website: http://www.realage.com/

My wife Terry and I took Dr. Roizen's quiz to determine our "Real Age". The quiz covers a wide variety of **lifestyle questions**, each of which either adds to or subtracts from your chronological age. Mine came out to **minus 16** (making my "Real Age" 52 at the time). My wife's came out to **minus 14** (making her "Real Age" 32 at the time). To take this quiz, just go to his website by clicking on the link above.

Dr. Roizen has an extended discussion on antioxidants (Vitamin C, E, etc.) and their role in controlling the **"free radicals"** which damage the genes in your cells.

It is pretty clear from all the research I have done that most cancers can be prevented by proper **diet, supplements and exercise**. Each of these three can be visualized as a leg on a **three-legged stool.** If any one is neglected, the stool collapses – your body degenerates and you get sick. We will cover supplements and diet guidelines in this chapter. Diet and exercise are the subjects of "booklets" which accompany this book.

[NOTE: Many people have pointed out to me their view that this "stool" actually has a fourth leg. They say it is our **spiritual nature** and its positive effect on our health. I will not try to influence you one way or another on this subject.]

Treating Your Cancer

In summary, **CANCER IS NOT A "DISEASE."** It is simply your body's own cells which have assumed an **abnormal function** as a result of damage to their normal functioning. Stem cells multiply much more rapidly than cancer cells…so cancer cells are not even the most **rapidly dividing** cells in your body. They're just abnormal cells that need to be brought under control.

Your body produces cancer cells **every day**, by the millions. Your normal cell policing mechanism takes care of them – until it can't any more. Then you are eventually diagnosed with cancer.

Your cancer probably **took years to develop** to the point where it can be detected. If you need a cause, blame it on your lifestyle. With that understanding, you also know that treating cancer is a

lifelong process. Once you have the cancer under control, or in "remission," which usually only takes a few weeks with my recommended regimen, you must continue to battle it with good lifestyle choices and support for your immune system for the **rest of your life.**

You can look on cancer as a **chronic condition,** something like hypertension (high blood pressure), heart trouble or diabetes. You must keep your body in top-notch cancer fighting shape. You **cannot** just revert to your old lifestyle and expect the cancer to stay away.

It's Baaaaack!

Unfortunately, **when cancer recurs**, because it was not kept under control, it tends to metastasize (spread) **more aggressively.** But, don't worry. In Chapters 5 and the bonus books on Diet and Exercise, I'm going to show you exactly how to avoid this.

Conventional cancer treatment (surgery, chemotherapy and radiation) **destroys your immune system**. Oncologists pay little attention to rebuilding it or changing your lifestyle. This is why cancer patients treated with conventional treatment seem to get better, only to have the cancer **recur** in a few months or years in a more aggressive form.

The succeeding chapters in this book will deal **in detail** with specific options available to every cancer patient. Many of these are supported by major research efforts. Many of them have spawned **groups of survivors** that have formed to get the information to other cancer sufferers.

In **Appendix A, Resources Summary**, is a complete list of the resources you can use to find more detail than I can include in this book. Also, the web sites will allow you to keep up-to-date on new developments as they occur, as will my newsletter.

Cancer Prevention

Many of the anti-oxidants our body needs to gobble up the free radicals and prevent cancer **must come** from supplements. If you've talked to your doctor lately about this subject, you were probably not encouraged by his response. Most physicians feel that supplements are **unnecessary**. A "proper" diet will provide all the vitamins, minerals, enzymes you need, they say. Just eat a "balanced" diet.

One prolific author on cancer – its treatment and prevention -- is **Ralph W. Moss, PhD**. Dr. Moss has written **13 books** on cancer therapy, causes, cures, prevention, etc., including *Questioning Chemotherapy, Herbs Against Cancer* and *The Cancer Industry*. This excerpt is from one of his books, published in 2000, called **Antioxidants Against Cancer.**

"Attitudes of Doctors

Thousands of scientific articles point to the power of antioxidants, yet many doctors are not taught about this in medical school. Others may know about this exciting development but shy away from it because they fear peer pressure or stigmatization. And all too often, doctors respond to positive reports with a warning that patients should not take food supplements.

The conventional line is that research is promising, but there just isn't enough data on which to base firm conclusions...

Certainly, few medical interventions can have less risk than eating a diet high in antioxidants. We are not talking about *taking arsenic here, but about **brightly colored fruits and vegetables**, as well as concentrated extracts. Yet many physicians draw the line when you discuss antioxidants and say, '**Much too risky. Not enough known.**'*

*No wonder lay people are turning to books, magazines, and Websites for information on antioxidants, and that many patients **hesitate to even discuss** questions of nutrition with their doctor. Patients are becoming more educated **(sometimes more educated than their doctors!)** and more empowered."*

If you would like to read more of Dr. Moss's work, these excerpts are from his book *"Antioxidants Against Cancer"*, copyright 2000, by Ralph W. Moss, Ph.D. You may also want to visit his website: http://www.CancerDecisions.com.

Effective Antioxidant Supplements

We've been talking about **antioxidants** in relation to cancer prevention. They are also important in the prevention of heart attacks, strokes, macular degeneration of the eye, and about **one hundred other illnesses** associated with aging.

The reasons for including antioxidant-rich foods and supplements in your daily routine go **far beyond cancer**.

Let me give you here the best source for a **supplement** that covers all the bases. If you know of a better one, I'd like to hear about it. Please send me an e-mail at: uhealcancer@gmail.com.

For just **over 18 years**, I have been receiving a newsletter called **"Alternatives"** written by **Dr. David G. Williams.** His writings about everything having to do with healthy living have been **immensely helpful** to my family and me.

[By the way, **nothing** I recommend in this e-book **results in even one dime of income** for me. I am truly writing this for your benefit, not for mine. If I **ever do get paid** for anything, it will be clearly marked as an ad.]

Dr. Williams has a very useful website. It now contains archive copies of his monthly newsletters, all the way back to 1985. This is a Mother Lode of health information. You can purchase for four or five dollars any of the back issues that interest you. Check it out at http://www.drdavidwilliams.com/.

About the antioxidants...Dr. Williams, in 1996, put together something he called **"Daily Advantage".** It is a little transparent plastic package containing 8 capsules. I take one package with breakfast and another with lunch or dinner, as Dr. Williams advises.

Here's how he describes the "Daily Advantage" nutrient package:

*"I've carefully chosen the **65** vitamins, minerals, antioxidants, herbs, superfoods, amino acids and digestive enzymes that are in Daily Advantage, based on all my **years of research** into nutritional supplementation.*

*...these hard-to-find nutrients work together to **supercharge the antioxidants** in the vitamin complex, making the overall formula more powerful and better able to destroy the **free radicals** attacking your cells."*

Here are the ingredients in each Daily Advantage set of capsules:

Essential Vitamins and Minerals:
- Vitamin A   5,000 IU
- Vitamin C   2,000 mg
- Vitamin D   800 IU
- Vitamin K   60 mcg
- Thiamine (Vitamin B1)   50 mg
- Riboflavin (Vitamin B2)   50 mg
- Niacin   126 mg
- Vitamin B6   110 mg
- Folic Acid   400 mcg
- Vitamin B12   100 mcg
- Biotin   300 mcg
- Pantothenic Acid   150 mg
- Calcium   1,000 mg
- Iodine   100 mcg
- Magnesium   500 mg
- Zinc   20 mg
- Selenium   200 mcg
- Copper   2 mg
- Manganese   10 mg
- Chromium   200 mcg
- Molybdenum   100 mcg
- Potassium   100 mg
- Vanadium   150 mcg
- Choline   100 mg
- Quercetin   50 mg
- N-acetyl cysteine   50 mg
- Trace Minerals Complex   50 mg
- Lemon Bioflavonoids   40 mg
- Para-aminobenzoic acid (PABA)   30 mg
- Inositol   100 mg
- Silica   26 mg
- Rutin (from buckwheat)   10 mg
- Hesperidin (from citrus peel)   10 mg
- Boron   1,000 mcg

Advanced Antioxidant Shield

- Vitamin A (as beta carotene)   15,000 IU
- Vitamin E   400 IU
- Tocotrienols (from rice)   20 mg
- Coenzyme Q10   10 mg
- Alpha-Lipoic Acid   10 mg
- Lutein (from marigolds)   6 mg
- Lycopene (from tomatoes)   6 mg

Herbal Superfood Booster

- Spirulina (from algae)   750 mg
- Turmeric (from root)   200 mg
- L-Taurine   200 mg
- Siberian Ginseng Root   180 mg
- Bee Pollen   100 mg
- L-Carnitine   100 mg
- Royal Jelly   50 mg
- Astragalus (from leaf)   50 mg
- Ginger Root   50 mg
- Gymnema Sylvestre   50 mg
- Pancreatin   50 mg
- Ox bile   50 mg
- Green Tea Extract   50 mg
- Siberian Ginseng Extract   50 mg
- Panax Ginseng Extract   40 mg
- Betaine Hydrochoride (HCL)   20 mg
- Ginkgo Biloba   10 mg
- Lipase   10 mg
- Cellulase   10 mg
- Maltase   10 mg
- Protease   10 mg
- Amylase   10 mg

In July 2002, Dr. Williams added an 8th capsule to the package at no extra charge. He calls it "EFA Advantage." It consists of several fish oil (mercury-free) extracts rich in Omega-3 fatty acids. Here is the composition:

- EPA (Eicosapertaenoic Acid)   100 mg
- DHA (Docosahexaenoic Acid)   150 mg
- Other Omega-3 fatty acids   50 mg
- Gamma Linolenic Acid   50 mg

You can get more information at his website or by calling **Mountain Home Nutritionals** in Ranson, West Virginia, the people who distribute **Daily Advantage** for Dr. Williams. They can be reached at (800) 888-1415.

I recently read a book called "Comparative Guide to Nutritional Supplements" by Lyle MacWilliam, BSc, MSc, FP. Mr. MacWilliam had taken 500 of the nutritional supplements on the market in the U.S. and Canada. From comparing the ingredients in each, he came up with a list of the **"100 best,"** which he further narrowed down to the **"top 5."** With the help of seven nutritionists, he also developed what he called a **"blended standard."** He describes this standard as "a nutritional benchmark we have created based on the independent recommendations of seven scientific authorities." This standard was used as the basis for comparison.

The book is interesting and I recommend it to you if you're a student of nutrition. The "Daily Advantage" described above was **not** one of the 500 products covered in this book. Naturally, I was curious. I compared the above ingredients with the "blended standard" in this book. I'm sure it won't surprise you that I found it was **"better than the best"** of the **"top 5."**

I pay about **$45 monthly** for Daily Advantage, including shipping by Priority Mail. I cannot even imagine how much it would cost me to buy these ingredients at the local health food store. I attribute my glowing health largely to this product, a **sensible diet** and **regular exercise**. I don't smoke. I drink very moderately (less than one glass of wine or equivalent per day).

Vitamin B or Not to B

I can't tell you how many lists I have read of vitamins, minerals, amino acids, etc. like the one above and **what each does for my body**. Have you done that? Doesn't each one make your **eyes glaze over**? They sure do mine.

To this day, I have **no idea** why it is good for me to eat some choline, quercetin, astralagus or ginger root each day. If a gun were held to my head, I **could not** tell you what all of Dr. Williams' **69 ingredients** do for me...or what dire results would threaten my body if one were eliminated.

The **exceptions** are the **antioxidants** -- which include Beta-carotene, Vitamin E, tocotrienols, coenzyme Q10, alpha lipoic acid, lutein and lycopene. These I have studied enough to **know why** they are good. They are the best thing you can take to **prevent cancer** and lots of other **degenerative diseases**. Also, I know that **Vitamin C** is great for your production of **collagen** that supports your joints, soft tissues, proper bone formation and prevents metastasis of cancer (see below). It also helps maintain **strong blood vessels**, your **immune system** and your body's own repair capabilities.

All I can tell you is that since beginning his **Daily Advantage** supplement program in 1996, I have had **no recurrence** of the many colds, flu and other maladies that I suffered through before

I started on it. This includes many years when I took Centrum Silver and many other "drugstore" supplements every day.

I have **lots of energy**, I **sleep well** and I enjoy **exercise**. I play 18 holes of **golf** twice a week (weather permitting), **sing** in a men's *a cappella* chorus and quartet and **play bridge** on the computer with people from all over the world. I was 76 in January, 2008.

After Antioxidants, What?

So, you've bought Dr. Williams **Daily Advantage** or whatever you think is better and you're **taking it every day.** Is that all? Not quite.

Ultra-Fit

The doctor most directly responsible for my gaining control over my health is **Dr. Joe Davis.** I met him at one of his Ultra-Fit "wellness" centers in San Antonio in 1992. I was 60 years old and in pretty sad shape.

Dr. Davis is an **internal medicine** specialist. He also is a **human being** who has fought through **obesity** and **alcoholism** to become a competitive weight lifter and founder of multiple Ultra-Fit centers around the country.

His book "Ultra-Fit" and the wellness centers were the result of his working with **thousands of patients** over a span of **15 years**, most of whom were obese and out-of-shape. Let me quote from Dr. Davis's book "Ultra-Fit" along with **my comments.**

*"It is my personal belief, as a physician of internal medicine, that **dietary factors** serve as the principal cause of our **most***

common killers *in the United States. The consequences of eating* ***too much fat*** *result in huge, staggering, burdensome* ***problems.*** *It costs society* ***billions and billions*** *of dollars each year to stem fat-related diseases.*

I am not over-dramatizing fat-related illnesses. Sure, ***other factors*** *figure into the equation that triggers* ***any one*** *of these illnesses.*

However, simply because you carry ***excess fat*** *on your body you* ***increase your chances*** *of developing one of these illnesses in your lifetime. The* ***longer*** *you carry excess fat, the* ***greater*** *your chances.*

The human animal has ***evolved genetic machinery*** *for conserving and* ***storing calories as fat*** *during intermittent periods when food is lacking. Only since the twentieth century have we developed the technology for food production, storage, and distribution so that, for practical purposes, we* ***no longer suffer from a lack of food*** *-- or at least not in the affluent parts of the world.*

Think about that. For millions of years, man constantly ***searched for food***, *suffered famines. Suddenly, in the last* ***fifty years***, *the United States suffers from* ***excess*** *food production.*

It takes ***work not to become fat*** *in America!"*

Where To From Here?

Free radicals are **bad**. Bad fats cause **more**. What do we do about it? Dr. Davis prescribed **changes in lifestyle** – diet, exercise and even mental images. He cited hundreds of examples of how his patients applied these ideas.

Will it work for you? Probably. Several "booklets" are included in the back of this book. In the first two, **"Stop Your Aging With Diet;"** and **"Stop Your Aging With Exercise;"** I will cover in detail how I have applied the ideas of Dr. Davis and other physicians and therapists.

Now, we will turn to your most immediate concern – "How do I put this knowledge to work to **heal** my (or my loved one's) cancer?" Please read on.

CHAPTER 4
TREATING YOUR CANCER

"As a chemist trained to interpret data, it is incomprehensible to me that physicians can ignore the clear evidence that **chemotherapy** *does much, much* **more harm than good**.*"*
Alan C. Nixon, Ph.D., Past President, American Chemical Society

The Basics

Cancer patients regularly **endure** treatments that are every bit as **barbaric** as the "bleeding" treatment used by doctors in the 15th century. Why? The answer lies in the **"politics" of cancer**.

If chemotherapy or radiation of any kind has been suggested for you or anyone you know or love, you **MUST** do some reading on your own and form your own opinion. I saw my former wife's body slowly **tortured and destroyed** by "chemo cocktails" over **four long years**. It reduced her to a **scrawny, pain-wracked invalid** without, in my judgment, extending her life by **even one day**.

Let's take a closer look at the **"conventional"** cancer treatments -- surgery, chemotherapy and radiation, also called **"debulking"** therapies.

Surgery

If you have one of the most common forms of cancer -- breast, prostate, colon, lung, etc. -- a **"hard" tumor** is usually found.

This is a characteristic of about **90% of the cancers** reported every year. At some point, your oncologist or surgeon is going to suggest **removing it**. Marge had it done several times.

The reading I have done suggests that frequently the **surgical removal** of the tumor often **causes metastasis** that may not have occurred. You will be worse off for having the surgery, even if you recover fully from the surgery.

The surgeon will say, as he did to me, **"We got it all."** He will **always be wrong.**

A cancer tumor the size of the eraser on a pencil contains a **billion** cancer cells. If only a few of these individual rascals escape the surgeon's knife, **as they always do**, your cancer is very likely to recur, unless you carefully rebuild your immune system.

The statistics say that if a tumor is found **"early,"** it will only reappear 50% of the time. With what we know about cancer statistics, I would expect this one to be **optimistic**. But, let's accept it. You have a **50/50 chance** that you will be just as bad off **after the removal**. Plus, you have **some chance** that you will be **much worse off**, because metastasis will occur.

Nevertheless, surgical removal of a tumor is **often desirable**. The "debulking" it offers will often bring the number of cancer cells down to a point where your body's own immune system can **"mop up"** the remaining cancer cells. This is true, however, only if you adopt a **strict regimen** to rebuild your immune system.

As we will see shortly, there are 350 treatments with natural substances which all have **evidence** that they successfully treat some __terminal__ cancer patients and many cancer tumors. Please

explore some of them before you turn your care over to a surgeon, oncologist or radiologist.

Each of these treatments shows **positive results within weeks**, results that can be detected with conventional methods -- MRI, CT scan, PET scan and blood tests. Depending on the stage of your cancer, you may want to try them before, during, after **or instead of** your "conventional" treatment. If your cancer doctor won't discuss this intelligently with you, **please** find another doctor.

Chemotherapy

For the purposes of this discussion, we will refer to chemotherapy as the **poisoning** of dividing cells using **cytotoxic drugs**. That's what chemotherapy is.

There are lots of other drugs used in cancer treatment to manage adverse reactions to the poison; alter hormonal balance; modify biological responses; or boost the immune system (interferon, etc.). For simplicity, we will not discuss those.

Chemotherapy uses various combinations of **toxic drugs** to poison cells as they divide. Remember the number **75 trillion**? That's the number of cells in the average person's body. **Each day, 29 billion or so** of these replace themselves by division. The cancer cells are dividing to form new malignant cancer cells. **Billions** of healthy cells are also **dividing every day** to replace themselves.

The chemotherapy "cocktails" **cannot distinguish** between cancer cells and healthy cells. They **bombard** them all with the same napalm. Ever wonder why almost all chemotherapy patients **lose their hair**? Guess where some of the **fastest dividing cells** in your body are? You guessed it. They're in your hair. **Not cancer cells**, just healthy cells replacing themselves. But there are lots more in your intestines and other vital organs and in your bone marrow. **Blast them all!** That's why all chemotherapy patients **feel like hell** and most **wish they were dead**! Marge sure did.

Does this strike you as **barbaric treatment**? Wouldn't you be looking for **anything but** this way to "treat" your patients if you were an oncologist? Most of them are well meaning but **caught up in the system**. The **drug money** (much of it involved in chemotherapy) drives the system. Most of the people doing the **alternative research**, at least in the U.S., are **not practicing cancer doctors** (oncologists). The research the cancer doctors and their paid "flunkies" at research centers do is **almost totally** funded by the **drug industry**.

There are **a few malignancies** that are **highly responsive** to chemotherapy. In October 1971, Dr. Gordon Zubrod, , a leader of the National Cancer Institute, presented a list of these. All of these are **rare in adults**. But, most important, the list **has not changed** since 1971. Here it is:

Burkitt's lymphoma; Choriocarcinoma; Acute Lymphocytic Leukemia; Hodgkin's Disease; Lymphosarcoma; Embryonal Testicular Cancer; Wilms' Tumor; Ewing's Sarcoma; Rhabdomyosarcoma; Retinoblastoma.

That's it. In the 37 years since that list was published, there is **no solid evidence** that chemotherapy for the other, more common, cancers results in **significant increased survival**. There is plenty of evidence that the chemotherapy is **carcinogenic** (causes other cancers).

I would not rule out using chemotherapy, particularly if I had one of the rare types of cancer listed above. One of **my daughters** had Wilms' Tumor when she was **three**. Removal of the affected kidney and chemotherapy **saved her life** and she had no recurrence.

You, too, may know someone who has had their cancer go into "remission" after treatment with chemotherapy drugs. They are among the lucky ones. But, please **consider** other gentler alternatives before you accept "high dose" chemotherapy.

Remember, time is usually **not critical** in treating cancer. It has taken years to develop to the point where it is detected. You certainly have **weeks, at the very least,** to overcome it.

Approach chemotherapy with a very skeptical attitude. Most of the time you don't have to subject yourself or your loved one to this **medieval form of "treatment."**

Consider that since 1971 when the "War On Cancer" started, about **$2 trillion** (with a "t") has been spent on conventional cancer treatment and research. Yet, despite the government and private sector's work to put a positive face on cancer survival rates, they **have not improved**. The latest statistics show more Americans dying from common cancers than ever before. For example, the January 10, 2002 issue of the *New England Journal of Medicine* stated that 20 years of clinical trials using chemotherapy on advanced lung cancer have yielded survival improvement of **only two months**.

According to an article in the January, 2003 issue of *Life Extension, "the institutions we have counted on to find a cure (National Cancer Institute, American Cancer Society, drug companies, etc.) have failed. This is not an allegation, but an admission made by the National Cancer Institute itself."*

Knowledge is power. If your doctor won't cooperate with you in experimenting with some of the treatments we will discuss, you should **get another doctor**. (See the list of resources for finding one in Chapter 1 above.)

Radiation

The third "approved" method of treating cancer is **radiation therapy.** If you have cancer, the subject **will come up.** For certain cancerous tumors, radiation is effective in **reducing the size** of the tumor. Most of the time the side effects are significant and very harmful. Once again, radiation **does not distinguish** between **cancer cells** and **normal cells**.

Cancer is a "systemic" condition. Your whole body is involved. **Reducing the tumor size** does not equate to **curing the cancer**. Why risk the side effects (including other cancer tumors) of radiation when treatments which deal with your whole body's cellular metabolism with no risk are readily available?

If you are considering either chemotherapy or radiation, you should definitely read a book called *Antioxidants Against Cancer,* by Ralph W. Moss, Ph.D., copyright 2000, published by Equinox Press, Inc. and available at amazon.com, Barnes & Noble, etc.

Dr. Moss is familiar to you if you've read everything in this book. His **ten previous books** cover the waterfront of cancer therapy. This one, however, gives a very close look at the **importance of antioxidants**. They are vital for both fending off cancer and other disease and for **tolerating** better both **chemotherapy and radiation**.

More importantly, he points out that patients who have had chemo or radiation **never recover** the antioxidant levels in their bodies without appropriate supplements. These antioxidants are

vital to life. He discusses each supplement in depth and how various chemo drugs and radiation affect it.

Insulin Potentiation Therapy (IPT)

There are many options available to you. If you are still considering conventional chemotherapy or radiation in any form, here is some detail on an option. You will probably not hear about this from your oncologist. It is something you must consider, however, because it is much more effective than the normal "high dose" chemotherapy and results in **far fewer side effects**. It is called Insulin Potentiation Therapy (IPT).

What Is It?

During Insulin Potentiation Therapy a small dose of insulin is given to the patient that induces a state of low **blood sugar (hypoglycemia)**. When the patient begins to have symptoms such as a feeling of lightheadedness and weakness (hypoglycemia symptoms) [usually in about 30 minutes], low doses of traditional chemotherapy are given intravenously. The insulin **tricks the cancer cells** into thinking food is coming. Their receptors open up. At that point, much smaller doses of chemotherapy is needed to kill the cancer cells. In other words, this treatment is **much more effective** than high dose chemotherapy. One study using methotrexate (a common chemotherapy drug) showed IPT to be 10,000 times more effective than high dose chemotherapy.

Another major advantage is that the patient retains much more energy to apply other healing methods. Here is a quote from one of the IPT web sites below:

"Conventional chemotherapy treatment can be so taxing that patients won't even consider, let alone take action on, other

cancer-fighting measures such as diet modification, exercise and meditation."

IPT vs High-Dose Chemotherapy

The main advantage of IPT is the reduction in side effects. The most common side effect from IPT is fatigue during the day of treatment. Rarely some nausea occurs.

As most of us have seen in our relatives and friends, the side effects of high dose chemotherapy can include suppression of the immune system, hair loss, nerve, heart, kidney, liver injury and, of course, death. Here are some facts about conventional high-dose chemotherapy that you'll never hear from your oncologist:

➤ It kills the P53 tumor-suppressor gene.
➤ It distorts the DNA of healthy cells, making them pre-cancerous and opening the door to future recurrences.
➤ It is a tightrope walk between how much chemo will kill the cancer before the chemo kills the patient.
➤ Cancers develop immunities to chemo drugs. This is why conventional oncologists have to move from one chemo drug to the next until they have to admit that "we've tried everything there is available and there is nothing more to do."
➤ If cancer recurs, it usually does so between 6-12 years after the initial diagnosis. Recurrence after high-dose chemo is a stronger cancer occurring in a weaker body. At that point, the cancer will have built-in immunities to most conventional chemo drugs.

But Does The IPT Work?

The results, as confirmed by several of my readers, can be **dramatically successful**. The small amounts and the reduced side effects have **healed them with minimal discomfort.** Obviously, nothing works for everyone and IPT is no exception.

Why doesn't your doctor know about this effective, less expensive, less damaging protocol? The FDA hasn't approved it, except as an **"experimental procedure."** Thus, some, but not all, insurance companies will pay for it. Medicare will not pay for it.

The National Cancer Institute (NCI) has had a researcher assigned to study it and do clinical trials since September 2000, but he has been given **no funding yet.** Don't hold your breath until he gets this money. You don't have to wait for the bureaucracy to get around to approving this procedure. IPT has been used very successfully to fight cancer for **over 78 years** and **it is legal**.

The Doctors Garcia – True Pioneers

Dr. Donato Perez Garcia, Sr. discovered IPT and began using it in Tijuana in 1930. Here are some **interesting statistics**. At the IPT course in Las Vegas, Nevada in February 2001, **Dr. Donato Perez Garcia** showed a slide of the "Morbidity" (bad outcomes) that his family (three generations of physicians) has had administering IPT.

Donato Perez Garcia, Sr., M.D. (ORIGINATOR OF IPT) (1896-1971)
YEARS OF DOING IPT 1930-1971: **41 YEARS MORBIDITY 0%**

Donato Perez Garcia Bellon, M.D. (1930-2000)

YEARS OF DOING IPT 1956-2000: **44 YEARS MORBIDITY 0%**

Donato Perez Garcia, Jr., M.D. (Still living)
YEARS OF DOING IPT 1983-2000: **17 YEARS MORBIDITY 0%**

The family of three physicians who founded IPT and have over 100 years of experience with it (there is some overlap in their careers), have never had a negative outcome **because of IPT**.

Why doesn't your oncologist know about this if it has been around for 78 years? It's not because it hasn't been documented to the cancer "system." In fact, IPT physicians have **briefed the National Institutes of Health** several times. There are **numerous published studies** in professional journals.

One obvious reason why it is not popular is the potential **loss of money** to the cancer industry. It is estimated that every cancer patient will produce **$800,000** to **$1,200,000** for the industry by the time he/she is given his or her last treatment. Such a simple, effective, and dramatic treatment that uses much less of the chemotherapy drugs would severely **cut into the industry's profits**. You do not have to be a victim of this evil greed.

To get smart quickly about this treatment and locate an IPT doctor near you, go to:

http://www.IPTforcancer.com

For some testimonials and other information about IPT, go to:

http://www.iptq.com or www.ElkaBest.org

The Cost

Several of my readers who have used this treatment in various parts of the country confirm that the cost is about **$13,000** for the initial three weeks of treatment (less at Dr. Garcia's clinic in Tijuana). It is done on an outpatient basis, but you need to stay in the vicinity of the clinic. While the IPT itself is normally done only twice a week, other treatments such as intravenous Vitamin C, immune system boosters, oxygen therapy, hyperthermia, etc. are done daily.

My Take On IPT

Before you seek out an IPT doctor, I suggest you think about the following. IPT is just one of the cancer treatments that concentrate on **killing cancer cells**. It is certainly more humane and effective than "high dose" chemotherapy. But remember, killing the cancer cells is **not how you recover from cancer**. You recover by rebuilding your body's balance and making it "hostile" to cancer cells. Once your body has its cancer-fighting balance restored, it takes care of the cancer cells, **just as it always had** before you were diagnosed with cancer.

Why spend money and time on treatments which just kill cancer cells? Why not focus your effort on **restoring your body's balance.** The self-treatment regimen I recommend in Chapter 5 of this book takes about 6 weeks to do that and **costs about $200**. Wouldn't it make more sense to try that first, before you seek out treatments which just kill the cancer cells and cost many times more? Think about it.

Selecting A Treatment – Some General Guidelines

- ➢ **Rarely** is treating the cancer an **"emergency"** decision. Take your time.

- ➢ Always focus your attention on restoring the **"environment"** in which the cancer cells live, not on killing the cancer cells.

- ➢ Before you spend a lot of **money and time** on cancer doctors, clinics and procedures, try the six-week diet and supplement regimen in Chapter 5 of this book.

- ➢ Don't accept **"response rate"** statistics. If the tumor "responds" to a particular treatment, that is counted as a plus by most oncologists. This is **irrelevant** to you, however. **5-year survival rates** are meaningless, also. What matters is the **quality of life** during and at the end of treatment and healing the cancer to the point where you live a normal lifespan and die of something else.

- ➢ If you don't have the energy to read about your options, **get an "advocate"** to do it for you and advise you.

- ➢ Avoid **"mainstream"** clinics and doctors – M. D. Anderson, Mayo Clinic, Sloan-Kettering Cancer Center, etc. The treatments you will receive there are never going to include the options you will read about shortly. Remember the American Cancer Society's "unproven remedies" list. None of the most prominent mainstream doctors and hospitals can stray far from conventional treatments – surgery, chemotherapy and radiation.

> Don't balk when your health insurance or Medicare **does not cover** the treatment you are considering. You are dealing with **your life** here. Nothing is more important than healing your cancer.

Testing Your Progress

When you choose a treatment, hopefully the regimen I outline in Chapter 5, you will want to know if it is working. Fortunately, there is an effective and inexpensive way to do that. It is described in detail in Chapter 5.

"Standard" Blood Tests

You've been having blood tests all your life. But did you realize that they are **full of vital information** for you about disease prevention?

Did you realize that your doctor probably has not given you any of that information -- probably because he/she doesn't know what it is?

A couple of years ago, I had a complete blood test performed at "Lab One" in San Antonio. It was unique in two ways. First, I ordered and paid for it myself **(no doctor's prescription required)** by calling the people at:

http://www.directlabs.com

Second, it was complete. 33 elements of blood chemistry tested. Most of the blood tests ordered by your doctor are **quite limited**. HMOs are very picky about what they will pay for. So, unless some diagnosis calls for it, many elements in the blood test are omitted because they add to the expense.

Ask the people at the lab where you get tested for a complete explanation of the results of your test. What you're looking for are **"sub-clinical" indicators**. The "normal" limits on most blood test results only show if you have a serious "clinical" problem.

Some important things to keep in mind:

1. Taking charge of your own health care includes understanding your blood tests.

2. Normal blood tests give you no clue about sub-clinical problems that can be dealt with before they become disease. Even if they did, your doctor is unlikely to know how to treat them -- except to treat the symptoms with some kind of prescription drug.

3. The "normal" blood test your doctor gives you is limited. Almost all doctors work under the "eagle eye" of an HMO. The more complete blood tests are more expensive. Draw your own conclusions.

4. Most degenerative "reactions" (like cancer, diabetes, arthritis, etc) have given clues in the blood chemistry long before medical doctors diagnose them. In most cases, they can be headed off by changes in diet and supplementation.

Live Blood Cell Analysis

This test may also be called a **"phase contrast lens"** study. A simple blood drop sample is taken and placed under a high-powered microscope. On a TV monitor, you will **see** the formations and activity of all your cells – red, white and platelets – floating around "live and in living color."

You and the doctor or nutritionist will be able to see whether they are functioning properly or if they are deficient or malformed and **what the cause is**. You will also see if you have a lack of enzymes, liver congestion, kidney congestion, fungal formations and **much, much more**.

This is one test that you will be able to **see for yourself** and not just get a result from your doctor's lab. The doctor will prescribe supplements, vitamins, herbs or minerals that are specific for the condition that this test shows. There is no magic to this test. It is very logical. It costs only **about $40.** Subsequent tests can be put on the same video tape, so you can easily compare them.

The **cost** of this test and treatment is in the **supplements**. But instead of the "hit and miss" approach most of us take to vitamins, herbs, enzymes and other supplements, you will be taking **those you specifically need** for your condition.

Any M.D., N.D. (naturopathic doctor) or nutritionist who has the equipment can do this test. Ask about it before you select your doctor or clinic.

Thyroid Panel T3, T4 and TSh

Your health insurance and Medicare cover this test. A **hyperactive or hypoactive thyroid gland** is one of the contributory factors to many major diseases or conditions such as heart disease, cancer, parasites, blood clotting and others. It is a simple blood test. There are homeopathic and naturopathic remedies for low functioning or over-functioning thyroids.

Trace Mineral Test

This test costs about $150 and **may be paid for** by your health insurance or Medicare. Your blood sample is sent to a lab such as Metatrix in Norcross, Georgia. There are others that can do it. It takes about a week to get the results. The **profound importance** of this test is that it reads and outlines every mineral in your body. Heavy metals such as zinc, aluminum and iron where an excess can cause a problem are shown. Mercury leaching from **fillings in your teeth** will show up. Deficiencies in needed minerals such as manganese, selenium, magnesium, etc. are shown. Your naturopath or Medical Doctor can then recommend specific supplements, vitamins or herbs for your condition.

Natural Killer Cell Activity Test

This test (sometimes called a "four-hour radioactive-chromium release assay") determines the degree of strength of your Natural Killer (NK) cells. As we will see in the next section, **NK cell activity** is an indicator of the ability of your immune system to "mop up" cancer cells. At present, I know of two labs that perform this test:

Tiburon Diagnostic Laboratories
802 E. 16th St.
Tucson, AZ 85719
(877) 842-8766

Specialty Laboratories
2211 Michigan Ave.
Santa Monica, CA 90404-3400
(800) 421-7110

Anti-Malignin Antibody in Serum (AMAS) Test

This is advertised as the "most accurate cancer test in the world." It can detect cancer nearly **two years before** any other method now in use with accuracy **above 99%.** Even more important, it can accurately detect the **recurrence** of cancer – any form of cancer – long before other cancer "marker" tests, with far fewer false positives.

Most doctors are unaware of this test. It is not marketed like other, much more expensive, tests such as PET scans, CT scans, etc. It is performed only at the lab owned by the couple that discovered the antibody in 1974. They have patented the test. Any doctor can order it from Dr. Bogoch's Oncolab, 36 The Fenway, Boston, MA 02215, (800) 922-8378. The cost: $135 plus overnight shipping.

No one test is perfect. In the case of the AMAS test, it doesn't work for advanced cancer cases. The antibody it tests for is not there. Also, there have been cases of false negatives reported, **particularly for breast cancer**. Apparently, these occur with tumors larger than 5cm. However, I would strongly recommend that you discuss this test with your doctor. If your doctor is not interested, you can order the test kit and information yourself and find another doctor to prescribe it for you. One of my readers in Montreal did just that for his wife. Just call (800) 9CATest.

In my opinion, the HCG Urine Test described in Chapter 5 is superior to the AMAS test. It costs less, too.

How Often To Test

Even a healthy person should have these tests done once a year. Whatever they cost can easily be made up by **targeting your supplements** to your specific condition instead of guessing at dosages. If you have cancer, the HCG urine test (see Chapter 5) should be done **every two months**. The live blood cell analysis should be done **monthly.** The Natural Killer Cell Activity Test, which is quite expensive, the trace mineral test and the thyroid test should be done only as required by your doctor. The

AMAS test kit has guidelines for how often to test. If you do the HCG Urine test described in Chapter 5, you will not need the AMAS blood test.

Don't Panic

Above all, **don't panic** at your cancer diagnosis. A cancer diagnosis, no matter how severe, is **not a death notice**. Many thousands of people who have had severe, Stage IV metastasized cancer are **completely well today**. You can be, too. The treatment methods and tests in this book will give you your health back.

Whether you are the patient or caregiver, when your experience with cancer is over, you will have **learned many valuable lessons** about lifestyle that will help you live a long and happy life. Count your blessings!

Your Rights As A Patient

Sometimes I think the word patient was applied to us innocent users of the medical "system" because we are so.....patient. As a cancer "patient," it will pay you to be **IM**patient. As a cancer **advocate** for a friend or loved one, it will serve you well to be **even more impatient** than the patient.

Nothing will be more important in the initial days after your diagnosis than **knowing your rights** as a patient. Here is an excerpt from another book by Dr. Ralph W. Moss. Published in 1995, the book is called **"Questioning Chemotherapy."**

*"Consider this sage advice from a cancer patient's widow, who wrote to **The Cancer Chronicles** (11/93):*

*'**Question** your doctor. Question him **every step of the way**. The more serious the condition, the more serious the treatment, the **more stringent the questioning** must be. If you don't have the energy, enlist the help of someone who does.... **Don't be afraid to fight**. Question your doctor, the same way you would a politician, for the two are not dissimilar. If your doctor won't answer the questions, **find one that will**.... There is a **party line** within the medical system. Question your doctor. **Always.'***

*And indeed, **some doctors** welcome intelligent dialogue, and **appreciate** the chance to share the **complexities of their science** with inquisitive patients. Others don't. If a doctor gets angry, condescending, or evasive, it may be **time to look for another doctor**. Never allow yourself to be hustled. Most likely you pride yourself on being a **knowledgeable consumer** in the general marketplace. Be an **informed medical consumer**, as well.*

*You now have a yardstick by which to **measure the effectiveness** of cancer treatments. If a drug or regimen has not been **proven to cure**, significantly **prolong actual survival**, or improve the **quality of life** -- if it only temporarily shrinks tumors, with a probable loss in well being -- then it is at most entirely **experimental and unproven**, and should not be represented as anything else. At worst, it could be not just ineffective, but **painful, destructive -- even fatal**.*

*It may be time to look into other **alternative, nutritional, or nontoxic** treatments. It is my personal opinion that the **best of these treatments** are based on more plausible theories and **offer more compelling evidence** than most chemotherapy; they certainly do **far less harm**.*

*Patients and their loved ones are often understandably **devastated** when they learn that they have cancer. It is an*

additional blow *to learn that chemotherapy is **not likely to help**, much less cure. But cancer is **not a death sentence**. It can be a **turning point**.*

*The **loss of illusions** may be the **beginning of wisdom**."*

Some More Doctors' Opinions

Here are some quotes from doctors who I respect:

"We have a multi-billion dollar industry that is killing people, right and left, just for financial gain. Their idea of research is to see whether two doses of this poison is better than three doses of that poison."

Glen Warner, M.D., oncologist

"I look upon cancer in the same way that I look upon heart disease, arthritis, high blood pressure, or even obesity, for that matter, in that by dramatically strengthening the body's immune system through diet, nutritional supplements, and exercise, the body can rid itself of the cancer, just as it does in other degenerative diseases. Consequently, I wouldn't have chemotherapy and radiation because I'm not interested in therapies that cripple the immune system, and, in my opinion, virtually ensure failure for the majority of cancer patients."

Julian Whitaker, M.D.

"There have been many cancer cures, and all have been ruthlessly and systematically suppressed with a Gestapo-like thoroughness by the cancer establishment. The cancer establishment is the not-too-shadowy association of the American Cancer Society, the leading cancer hospitals, the National Cancer Institute and the FDA. The shadowy part is the

fact that these respected institutions are very much dominated by members and friends of members of the pharmaceutical industry, which profits so incredibly much from our profession-wide obsession with chemotherapy."

Robert C. Atkins, M.D., author, "Dr. Atkins New Diet Revolution" and founder, The Atkins Center in New York

"My studies have proved conclusively that untreated cancer victims live up to four times longer than treated individuals. If one has cancer and opts to do nothing at all, he will live longer and feel better than if he undergoes radiation, chemotherapy or surgery."

Professor Hardin B. Jones, Ph.D., University of California

"Everyone should know that the 'war on cancer' is largely a fraud, and that the National Cancer Institute and the American Cancer Society are derelict in their duties to the people who support them."

Linus Pauling, Ph.D., two-time Nobel Laureate

Now, for some specific self-treatments that I recommend you begin **immediately,** please read on.

CHAPTER 5
CANCER SELF-TREATMENTS THAT I RECOMMEND

"All of my knowledge is learned by standing on the shoulders of geniuses." Albert Schweitzer

Please don't feel you are exploring **uncharted territory** when you begin to treat your cancer with **"alternative"** treatments. In 1997, the recorded number of visits to alternative practitioners in the U.S. surpassed the number of visits to allopathic (conventional) physicians. That number has been rising ever since. A recent survey by Life Extension Foundation found that **80%** of cancer patients take one or more "alternative" treatments and **half of them** do not tell their doctor about these treatments. That is **not** what I recommend for you.

In this section of the book, I will describe cancer treatments that you need to **discuss with your doctor**, no matter who he/she is. However, if your current doctor is **not sympathetic** to these treatments, **start them anyway** while you look for one who is. They are treatments for which a **vast library** of information is available. They have been proven over many years to work on all types of cancer.

I will discuss in detail the ones I would adopt **if I had cancer**. What type of cancer? It wouldn't matter. Whatever type and stage of cancer I was diagnosed with, I would do the same things described here.

I will give you **the exact regimen** I would follow. It is not expensive. In fact, part of it costs nothing. Is it difficult? No, because I do most of it now for prevention. I know lots of people who have done this exact regimen and are "cancer-free" now. In fact, I know people who have healed themselves using just one of these six treatments. Guaranteed to work? Sorry. **No guarantees**.

You must research these beyond the information in this book. I'll give you resources to do that. Do this research **before** you discuss them with your doctor. In that way, you will be in a position to judge his/her reaction when you bring up the subject. **Don't just "ask your doctor"** about them. Very few doctors are as knowledgeable about these cancer treatments as you will be in a few minutes. Before you bring these up, you must be **thoroughly** convinced of their efficacy.

Immune System Boosters

Cancer and the Immune System

No cancer either begins or thrives if the patient's immune system is strong. So, a first priority for either prevention or healing is to get your **immune system** in **cancer-fighting shape**. Supplements are essential. We'll discuss diet later, but no diet should be considered adequate to reverse cancer. All require supplementation. Fortunately, you have many options. I will give you my first choice, and then discuss some of the options.

Beta-1,3D Glucan

Here is an article I published in the February 27th, 2007 edition of my newsletter.

"Those of you who have been reading my scribbling for awhile know I have always recommended the best immune system booster product I could find. Because there are so many options

for this essential function, I'm always open to new information. Well, last Saturday (3 days ago) I got hit squarely between the eyes with the most dramatic information on this subject I've ever heard. You REALLY need to pay attention to this one.

About a week ago, my biological dentist friend, Dr. John Tate of Spartanburg, South Carolina, suggested I contact Marilyn Becker of Transfer Point in Columbia, SC and get some information on their Beta-1,3D Glucan product. Dr. Tate knows I counsel a lot of cancer patients. In fact, I've referred several of them with root canal and other dental issues to him.

I called Marilyn and she said they happened to have an opening in the all-day seminar they were doing for some health care professionals and some of their newer distributors on Saturday, February 24th. She invited me to come down and sit in. I am very glad I accepted Marilyn's kind invitation.

The speaker that day was A. J. Lanigan. A. J. attended pharmacy school at the University of South Carolina from 1971 until 1975. For about the last 25 years, he has studied the immune system. He knows this complex subject better than anyone I have ever met or read. That puts him ahead of some elite company -- Dr. Mamdooh Ghoneum, , Dr. Richard Kinsolving, Dr. Hulda Clark, Dr. Michael Roizen, Dr. David Williams, Dr. Robert Rowen and many more.

With his vast knowledge of how this complex system works, A. J. has perfected a product which has the optimum effect in strengthening the immune system's efficiency without causing it to 'overcook' and trigger auto-immune responses. If you are a cancer patient or caregiver, this should be your absolute number one priority. No cancer patient has ever recovered until they have gotten their immune system back in shape.

What A. J. has done, which no other manufacturer of this type of product has ever done, to my knowledge, is encouraged institutions all over the country to study his product -- Beta-1,3D Glucan -- and compare its effectiveness with any of the other competitive products. These institutions include Harvard, Tulane, University of Louisville, Baylor, Johns Hopkins among others. What they have done, in many peer-reviewed studies, is shown that the particular product A. J. produces is far superior to all other immune system boosting products on the market. Yes, this includes RM-10 Ultra, the product I have been recommending most recently.

The products that have been tested and found wanting in relation to Beta-1,3D Glucan include BETAMax, Advanced Ambrotose by Mannatech, Immutol, Glucagel, Transfer Factor, Manopol, Maitake-Gold, MacroForce, Immune Builder, and dozens more. The rankings were based on in vivo experiments on animals by a major university in a side-by-side competitive assay.

You can learn a lot more about this product at the web site I'll give you and I encourage you to do so. At the discount prices you'll be offered, it costs about the same as RM-10 ULTRA. But let me give you a couple of the key facts I learned on Saturday.

> *Almost all immune booster products are soluble. That means that where they dissolve in the body and the effect they have as a result is difficult to control. Beta-1,3D Glucan is insoluble. It is a fiber-like substance. It gets where it belongs. Namely, it passes from the small intestine through the Peyer's patches to the lymphatic system. From there, it is carried into the blood stream, all the body's organs and even into the bone marrow by phagocytes (immune cells that gobble things). [Obviously, I am vastly over- simplifying this complex subject.]*

➤ *It "primes" the neutrophil immune cells to recognize cancer cells and kill them. These cells make up 50-60% of your immune system cells. Normally, they do not recognize cancer cells. Beta-1,3D Glucan binds to a receptor in the outer membrane of these cells. With this receptor activated, they "see" cancer cells as fungus cells and kill them. This adds these cells to your "army" of Natural Killer (NK) cells, macrophages, and lymphocytes. By the way, NK cells, macrophages and eosinophils also have glucan receptors making A.J.'s Beta 1,3-D glucan the single most effective immune modulator known.*

➤ *Taking the proper dose (depends on your weight) once a day on an empty stomach will double the effectiveness of your immune system. Because of the way it acts in your body, it is not necessary to spread these vegicaps through the day. Also, taking more will not produce any greater result.*

➤ *Beta glucan from mushrooms (like that in RM-10 ULTRA) and from cereal grains are much less effective than that from yeast like the Beta-1,3D Glucan from Transfer Point.*

An amazing video we saw (time-compressed, of course) showed that it took Natural Killer (NK) cells and macrophages over 52 hours to kill one melanoma cancer cell. Of course, this was in the body of a cancer patient with a relatively weak immune system.

To get complete information on this product and get the special discount they offer to you, my loyal readers just go to this special web site:

http://www.AboutBetaGlucan.com/bspecial

If you prefer, you can call Phyllis or Michael to place your order. Their toll-free number is (800) 746-7640. Outside the U.S., you can call (678) 560-1808. They are in the Atlanta area (Eastern Time).

Shipping in the U.S. is free.

[I probably need to remind newer readers that I make not a single dime from any product I recommend. No commissions, no affiliate status -- nothing. My only income from this project is from the sale of my book 'Cancer-Free' and from occasional fees for additional coaching.]

My wife and I have been taking this product since February, 2007 and you should, too. By the way, there is no harm to your system from taking the beta glucan extracted from yeast. Specifically, it does not cause yeast infections like *Candida albicans*, etc.

Phyllis and Michael sell another product which is very useful to cancer patients. It is an alkalizing, ionizing water filter for your drinking water. We keep ours set at a pH of **about 9.5,** which makes all the water we drink not only pure but very alkaline. Cancer patients have recovered by simply reversing the acid condition in their bodies. Take a look at this water filter. We love ours. You'll find the information at their other web site:

http://www.BetterWayHealth.com

MGN-3 (R.I.P.)

Before July 12th, 2004, I would have recommended MGN-3 here. Its power as an immune system stimulant was backed by **lots of scientific evidence**. Hundreds of my readers who have become cancer-free used it. Several used nothing else. In short, **it worked**. Too well, it seems. Pressure from Big Pharma finally succeeded. A frivolous lawsuit brought against Lane Labs by the FDA over labeling, begun in 1999, resulted in a decision by a New Jersey federal judge. On July 12th, 2004, he ordered Lane Labs, the only U.S. source for MGN-3, to shut down and reimburse everyone who had bought its products since 1999.

There are still routes to get MGN-3, but by now it has been overtaken by better (what I call **"second generation"**) immune boosting products like those above and below in this chapter.

If the kind of federal government nonsense such as that in the Lane Labs case makes you angry, as it should, you are **not powerless**. Frequently in my lifetime, movements by angry groups of voters have changed government policies. **You have a voice**. One group gaining strength is called "Campaign For Better Health." You can explore their movement and use their resources to contact your Congresspersons at:

http://www.BetterHealthCampaign.org

Another great foundation which deserves your support is the Natural Solutions Foundation. Their worldwide effort to protect your access to natural supplements is highly commendable. Check out their website and donate if you can. Go to:

http://www.HealthFreedomUSA.org

Other Options

Here are some other options to boost your immune system. I like to give you options. However, if you decide to use the **Transfer Point Beta Glucan** above, as I have, these are duplications and **not necessary.**

RM-10 Ultra

Sold at many web sites, this Garden of Life product is a combination of **10 different mushroom extracts** plus Folic Acid, Vitamin B12, Calcium and Selenium. This would be my second choice among the many options available for this purpose. I first noticed this product when several of my readers recommended it to me while I was still recommending MGN-3. RM-10 Ultra comes from Garden of Life, a source I trust.

There are no "therapeutic" doses for fighting cancer on the RM-10 bottle. See the paragraph on MGN-3 above for the reason. Actually, the FDA harassed Garden of Life about their labeling and I understand they had to change all their labels at great cost. At any rate, I would take **triple the "normal" dose on the bottle** if I had cancer. That works out to 6 capsules a day. A typical price (you should shop around) is $38 for 90 vegicaps plus shipping. At 6 capsules a day, that works out to about $90 a month. The Beta Glucan (see article above) is about $95-$125 per month for a therapeutic dose, depending on your body weight.

I would continue to take this dose for about 6 weeks, and then reduce it to the "maintenance" dose of 1 capsule twice a day ($30 per month). This is about the same cost as the maintenance dose of the Beta-1,3D Glucan described above. One web site which describes the contents of RM-10 Ultra is:

http://www.BeyondProbiotics.net/rm10ultra.htm

One of the things that caught my eye about RM-10 Ultra is that one of the mushroom extracts they use is **"agaricus blazei."** First discovered in Brazil, in a small village where no native had ever experienced cancer, this mushroom extract has been studied extensively by Japanese scientists. Japanese scientists are, without a doubt, the world's best when it comes to mushroom compounds.

The good news about this product is that it is effective at boosting the activity of both the **Natural Killer (NK) cells** but also the all-important **macrophage** (Greek for "Big Eater") cells of the immune system. Three of the mushroom extracts actually contain beta glucan, but as stated above, this is not as powerful as the beta glucan extracted from yeast.

Oncolyn

When I discussed this subject with a friend who owns a health food store in early 2001, she recommended I take a look at Oncolyn. She said it was **"better than MGN-3."** As with most supplements, there are indeed alternatives. I respect her opinion, so I did some research.

Like MGN-3 and RM-10 Ultra, Oncolyn **destroys cancer cells** and neutralizes the toxicity of most chemotherapy drugs. It also, however, acts as a **powerful anti-oxidant**, inhibits angiogenesis (which both delays tumor growth and suppresses tumor metastasis), and "induces differentiation of cancer cells back to normal cells."

Powerful stuff. It was formulated by Arthur H.K. DJang, M.D., Ph.D., M.P.H. He is a U.S. licensed physician and certified specialist by the American Boards of Pathology and the American Board of Nuclear Medicine with expertise in Infectious Diseases, Biochemistry and Immunology (Ph.D), Preventive Medicine (M.P.H.) and Cytopathology. Impressed? Me, too.

Oncolyn is totally **herbal and non-toxic**. You need to consult with your medical professional, but at the doses I have seen recommended for cancer patients, it is considerably more expensive than either the Beta-1,3D Glucan or the RM-10 Ultra.

Oncolyn is available at most health food stores and on the Internet. The best Internet source I've found is:

http://www.bellayre.com

The recommended "normal" dose of two per day costs $50 (60 capsules). However, a cancer patient should take triple this dose for at least the first six weeks, which makes the Oncolyn considerably more expensive than the others.

Why Are These First Priority?

Taking appropriate immune system boosting products will almost certainly **insure** that your cancer **will not recur**. Without this treatment, continued after you are declared "cancer-free," your cancer will **almost certainly recur** months or years after completion of your "debulking" therapy.

No instruments or tests today can detect the relatively small number of cancer cells that **always remain** after conventional treatment. Those cells are, by definition, the **hardiest**. With your immune system **destroyed by the chemotherapy**, radiation or surgery, they continue to divide in a **"cancer friendly"** environment.

If you or a loved one is diagnosed with cancer, immune system boosting is **PRIORITY ONE**. Best of all, this treatment is what is known as an **"adjunctive"** therapy. That means it does not require you to challenge your cancer doctor to approve an "alternative" treatment. With enough study of the available research, almost any respectable doctor should cheer you on in your use of these products. If he or she does not, **take them anyway**, and consider finding another doctor.

There are over 130 different types of cells in your immune system. One of the most important for cancer patients is the Natural Killer (NK) cell. There are billions of these in your body, but you can be assured that yours were not active enough or you would not have "gotten" cancer. The products described above activate your NK cells and make them rapacious killers of cancer cells.

Where's The Proof?

You may be wondering why I don't cite more scientific papers and "clinical" studies on the products I recommend. Basically, the reason is that nobody who sells a product that is in the "public domain" (i. e. that is able to be compounded and sold by anyone) can afford to spend the **$200-500 million** typically spent by drug companies to "test" a new synthetic drug.

Some of these products (MGN-3, Oncolyn, PolyMVA) are patented. That means they can be sold at a much higher price than those that are not patented. Price, in my experience, **does not correlate at all with efficacy**. In other words, you don't necessarily "get what you pay for."

Most of the "evidence" you'll find on the products mentioned in this book is what's called **"anecdotal."** Someone has tried it (usually **thousands of people**) and found that it worked. Is this good enough? Well, since almost all of these products are **harmless at any dose**, I'd say that's good enough to give them a try. It's your judgment call.

Are there scams in the "natural" health product business? **You bet**. Do all the "natural" health products have in them exactly what it says on the bottle? Sorry, **they don't**. In my opinion, your best insurance of getting an effective product is the **integrity of the source**. That's why I recommend sources like Transfer Point, Our Health Co-op, Garden of Life, and Green Supreme.

Actually, dozens of research papers on beta glucan (and other substances like antioxidants) are available on the Internet. If you are interested in an example, go to:

http://www.ncbi.nlm.nih.gov/PubMed/

Search for "glucan and macrophage." **Warning:** You will find the typical dense prose of research scientists in these papers, such as: *"Surface expression of phosphatidylserine on macrophages is required for phagocytosis of apoptotic thymocytes."* Maybe you'd just as soon take my word for it. [Chuckle!]

Flaxseed Oil & Cottage Cheese – The Budwig Diet

Following is a reprint of an article that appeared in my "Cure Your Cancer" newsletter on July 16th 2002. For the first and last time in over 8 years of publishing this newsletter, I **devoted the entire newsletter** to this subject. See if you agree with me on its pertinence to you or your loved one as an **effective and inexpensive** treatment.

In my research starting in 1998, I had run across Dr. Johanna Budwig, 's name several times. I always glossed over it when I heard her "formula" -- a little flaxseed oil mixed with cottage cheese.

Bad decision!!

Thanks to one of you, my faithful readers, I was introduced to the **FlaxseedOil2** chat group. More about them in a minute. Through this group's testimonials, I learned that this substance **UNIQUELY** kills cancer cells by the billions and makes every other cell in our body healthier – **at the same time**. Got your attention?

Since then, I have read many articles and books on this subject. It seems that there is **nothing like it in the world**. The cottage cheese is a perfect **carrier** for the oil. Once the flaxseed oil, with its high concentration of Omega 3 oil, gets to the cell wall (membrane), it surrounds it with little magnets which "suck in" oxygen. This oxidation of the cells has been recognized since 1931 as the primary way to make healthy cells healthier and kill cancer cells.

Here is a quote that I hope will rivet your attention on this topic.

An Oncologist Speaks

Dr. Dan C. Roehm, M.D., FACP, an **oncologist and former cardiologist** wrote an article in 1990 in the "Townsend Letter For Doctors & Patients." He said:

*"This diet is far and away the **most successful anti-cancer diet in the world**. What she (Dr. Johanna Budwig,) has demonstrated to my initial disbelief but lately, to my **complete satisfaction** in my practice is: **CANCER IS EASILY CURABLE**. The treatment is dietary/lifestyle, the response is immediate; the cancer cell is weak and vulnerable; the precise biochemical breakdown point was identified by her in **1951** and is specifically correctable, in vitro (test tube) as well as **in vivo (real).***

I only wish that all my patients had a PhD in Biochemistry and Quantum Physics to enable them to see how with such consummate skill this diet was put together. It is a wonder.

In 1967, Dr. Budwig broadcast the following sentence during an interview over the South German Radio Network, describing her incoming patients with failed operations and x-ray (radiation) therapy:

*'Even in these cases it is possible to restore health **in a few months** at most, I would truly say **90% of the time**.'*

*This has never been contradicted, but this knowledge has been a long time reaching this side of the ocean, hasn't it? Cancer treatment can be **very simple** and **very successful** once you know how. The cancer interests don't want you to know this.*

May those of you who have suffered from this disease (and I include your family and friends) forgive the miscreants who have kept this simple information from reaching you so long.

[signed] Dan C. Roehm, M.D. FACP"

Did you see that Dr. Roehm is an oncologist and cardiologist and a "Fellow of the American College of Physicians" (FACP)? His views are based on his own observations of patients in his practice. Also note that Dr. Budwig's 90% figure does **not include chemotherapy recipients**! Don't lower your odds by taking chemotherapy.

Here's another quote from a noted doctor:

*"A top European cancer research scientist, Dr Johanna Budwig, has discovered a **totally natural formula** that not only protects against the development of cancer but people all over the world who have been diagnosed with incurable cancer and **sent home***

to die *have actually been* **cured** *and now lead normal healthy lives.*

Robert Willner, M.D., Ph.D."

The Magic Bullet?

Have I abandoned my position that there is **no single cure** for all cancers? No. However, would I sit up and take notice of this particular treatment if I were you? Darn right! I hope you trust me enough by now to know that I would not emphasize anything to this extent unless I was **thoroughly convinced** that you should try it. I am eating it every day for prevention.

What Is It?

It's so simple that it seems ridiculous. After 30 years of research on fats and their effect on our cells, Dr. Budwig came up with **cottage cheese and flaxseed oil** as an effective preventative **AND HEALING MIXTURE** for cancer and many other ailments.

Flaxseed oil/cottage cheese, or **FO/CC** as it is referred to on the chat group, is very simple to prepare. You simply mix two-thirds cup of organic cottage cheese **(no preservatives)**, 1% or 2% fat, with **6 tablespoons of flaxseed oil**. Both ingredients are readily available at any health food store. This is the cancer patient's dose – **every day.** It can be divided in half to make it easier to eat it all. However, since it does oxidize, it should be eaten as soon as possible after it is mixed.

Organic yogurt (with live cultures) is a suitable substitute for cottage cheese (known as "quark" in Europe), according to Dr. Budwig. She says that using yogurt, you should **triple the amount**. In other words, use about 2 cups of yogurt with the 6

Eat alone – no other food when eating FO/CC

tablespoons of flaxseed oil. I know of no cancer patient who wants to eat this much of any one thing every day.

My wife and I add a packet of Stevia as a sweetener and some almonds, walnuts, strawberries, blueberries or all of the above. It makes a tasty "smoothie." These berries and nuts are cancer-fighting food, by the way.

Dr. Budwig says you can use a blender (pouring the FO/CC in **AFTER** it is well blended by hand). Then add the berries and nuts, but **not peanuts**.

I have found this mixture **so filling and full of protein** (the cottage cheese) for breakfast that I don't get hungry again until about 3 PM. As you'll see when we talk about the "cancer-fighting diet," this is a big plus. I have lots of energy. In fairness, I also eat a banana with it in the morning. One banana is about 29 grams of carbohydrate, so this is a **very filling breakfast**.

Why Does It Work?

The theory behind this odd combination? Dr. Budwig says the absence of **linoleic acids** in the average Western diet is responsible for the production of oxydase, which induces cancer growth and is the cause of many other chronic disorders. The use of oxygen in the body (one of the best ways to "erase" cancer cells) can be stimulated by **protein compounds of sulphuric content**, which make oils water-soluble and which are present in cheese, nuts, onion and leek vegetables such as leek, chives, onions and garlic, and **ESPECIALLY IN COTTAGE CHEESE.** _cold pressed (not heated)_

The flaxseed oil and the cottage cheese (or yogurt) must be **blended and eaten together** to be effective. They are synergistic. In other words, one triggers the healthful properties

For extra boost:
Supercharge results by adding 6 Tb. freshly ground flaxseed to blended FO/CC

98

ground flaxseed turns rancid after 15 min.

of the other. The cottage cheese loses all its dairy properties (casein, lactose, etc.) in this mixture. Dozens of people I know who are "lactose intolerant" eat this mixture every day with no adverse effects.

It is important to keep the oil in the refrigerator in the dark bottle it comes in after it is opened. Light and heat quickly make it rancid. I buy eight 12-ounce bottles at a time (about two months worth for my wife and me) from Barleans. They ship it directly to me, so it is **very fresh**. In over five years of use, I have had no problems with any rancid oil.

Special Program For Cancer Patients

If you have been diagnosed with cancer, you need to know about a special program at Barleans. They are, in my opinion, the **top quality manufacturer** of flaxseed oil. They also have a **special pricing program** for cancer patients. They currently sell it to the cancer patient at close to their wholesale price. All you have to do is call (800) 445-3529 (Pacific time). Believe me, with the price of this oil what it is in the health food store, this is a very generous program which you should take advantage of. Also, Barleans ships it directly to you the morning after the seeds are squeezed to make the oil. It is undoubtedly the **freshest oil** you can get.

So, you just eat the FO/CC mixture and wash it down with a Whataburger, french fries and a chocolate shake...**NOT!** As you might expect, the FO/CC is part of a lifestyle change that emphasizes food that is **not processed** and contains no "hydrogenated" anything. We will talk about the "no-noes" in a cancer-fighting diet later in this chapter.

Dr. Budwig's formula includes a **complete diet plan**, including a flax oil "spread," which can be used with fruits, vegetables, potatoes or grains such as rice, buckwheat or millet. It can also be added to sweet sauces and soups. There is also flax oil "mayo" which can be used for salads or healthy sandwiches.

I prefer to "keep it simple, stupid" (the old KISS principle). You may follow the complete Budwig diet if you like. All I can tell you is "What I would do if I were you." That's all I'm qualified to do. I would do the **FO/CC**. The rest of my diet would be as described later in this chapter.

If you would like to explore all the details on Dr. Budwig's diet and the "spread" and "mayo" recipes, just click on:

http://www.positivehealth.com/permit/Articles/Nutrition/turner60.htm

Or

http://www.BudwigVideos.com

More Science

In a book called "Oxygen Therapies" published in 1991, Ed McCabe offers this point of view on fatty acids:

*"The red blood cells in the lungs give up carbon dioxide and take on oxygen. They are then transported to the cell site via the blood vessels where they release their oxygen into the plasma. This released oxygen is 'attracted' to the cells by the 'resonance' of the 'pi-electron' oxidation-enhancing fatty acids. Otherwise, **oxygen cannot work its way into the cell**. 'Electron rich fatty acids' play a **decisive role** in respiratory enzymes, which are the basis of cell oxidation...*

*Don't eat anything hydrogenated **(like margarine or fried foods)** as it defeats oxygenation. Avoid products that say* *'hydrogenated.'*

*We should eat essential polyunsaturated fatty acids to enhance oxygenation. They can be found naturally in carotene, saffron, and **FLAXSEED OIL**.*" [Emphasis added.]

Dr. David Williams, one of my favorite health gurus, added four essential fatty acids (EFAs) to his Daily Advantage formula (see Chapter 3 above) in 2003. An article in his newsletter urges us to **drastically increase** our intake of **Omega-3** fatty acids, the exact formula of flaxseed oil.

Here's a quote from a "promo" I received on it from Dr. Williams in 2003:

"In case you haven't heard the great news, Dr. Williams just added a powerful, new Essential Fatty Acids (EFAs) complex to Daily Advantage. These EFAs, particularly the omega-3s, are critical for your cardiovascular system, cholesterol, blood pressure, brain function, immune system, joints, and just about every other system in your body."

Don't concern yourself with the difference between Omega-3, Omega-6 and Omega-9 fatty acids. Just realize that Omega-3's should be about **one to one** to Omega-6's in your diet for your body to work properly. The ratio of our "normal" diet today is **one or none** Omega 3 to **20 or 30** Omega 6.

Dr. Budwig's work has confirmed that this imbalance, caused by the "hydrogenated" fat in processed food, margarine, etc. is the cause of most infirmities we suffer from. Several studies have shown that our typical Omega-3 level in our bodies is **80% below normal**. The flaxseed oil, when mixed with cottage cheese or yogurt, restores that balance...period. End of scientific story.

...But Does It Really Work?

Being **skeptical** of any new idea that makes bold claims is **healthy**. When you have cancer, it is **essential**. I was quite skeptical of this treatment at first. I joined the chat group and pawed my way through the 20-25 e-mails a day. You may, of course, do the same, if you are so inclined. All you have to do is send a blank e-mail to:

FlaxseedOil2-subscribe@yahoogroups.com

Maybe I can save you a lot of trouble. After reading the messages of this group for about three weeks, I became thoroughly convinced that they are onto something significant for **ALL** cancer patients.

First, almost all of the participants are **recovering from cancer** and other diseases (strokes, diabetes, etc.). Second, all of them, without exception, are thoroughly convinced that their recovery is the result of the Dr. Budwig protocol. The founder of the chat group, **Clifford Beckwith**, was cured of **Stage IV prostate cancer** in the early 90's by Dr. Budwig's protocol. He was a **missionary** for this treatment until his death (not from prostate cancer) in 2006.

If you would like to read Cliff Beckwith's complete account of his experience, including dozens of other examples of **proper and improper** use of the FO/CC treatment, just go to:

http://www.beckwithfamily.com/Flax1.html

What Does It Treat?

Dr. Budwig's formula has been used therapeutically in Europe for prevention and treatment of: Cancer; Arteriosclerosis; Strokes;

Cardiac Infarction; Irregular Heartbeat; Liver (fatty degeneration); Lungs (reduces bronchial spasms); Intestines (regulates activity); Stomach Ulcers (normalizes gastric juices);
Prostate (hypertropic); Arthritis (exerts a favorable influence); Eczema (assists all skin diseases); Old Age (improves many common afflictions); Brain (strengthens activity); Immune Deficiency Syndromes (multiple sclerosis, autoimmune diseases such as lupus).

Some Testimonials

Here are some interesting testimonials.

Siegfried Ernst, M.D.

Seventeen years ago Dr. Ernst had developed cancer for which he had major surgery requiring removal of his stomach. Two years later he had a recurrence of the cancer and was offered chemotherapy as the only available remedy. There was little hope for survival as virtually all individuals with recurrence of this type of cancer rarely last a year.

Dr. Ernst knew that chemotherapy was not only ineffective for his type of cancer but completely destructive of the quality of life, so he refused. He turned to Dr. Budwig and her formula for help. He religiously followed Dr. Budwig's formula and fifteen years later has not had any recurrence of cancer. He is in perfect health and is tireless for a man in his late seventies.

Maria W.

Maria W. tells her story in her own words: *"I was told by the most expert of doctors that I would have to be operated on to cut out the cancerous tumor that was causing a swelling under my eye. They explained that the size of the tumor was much greater inside and that there was very serious bone involvement. The malignancy was too far advanced to respond to radiation treatment. The doctors planned to remove considerable facial tissue and bone. I was afraid for my life, but being a young woman, couldn't bear the thought of such disfigurement.*

When I heard about Dr. Budwig's natural formula, I was skeptical but desperate for help. After four months on this regimen, the swelling under my left eye completely disappeared. The doctors at the University hospital gave me many exhausting tests. One told me, 'If I didn't have your previous x-rays and medical history in front of me, I wouldn't believe that you ever had cancer. There is hardly any indication of a tumor remaining.' I never thought using Dr, Budwig's formula would be so successful. My whole family and I are very grateful."

Sandy A.

An examination of Sandy A. revealed arachnoidal bleeding due to an inoperable brain tumor. The doctors informed Sandy that he was beyond medical help. At his expressed wish, Sandy was discharged from the hospital and sent home to die in peace.

A friend brought Dr. Budwig's formula to Sandy's attention. Sandy writes:

"Since I went on the Budwig regimen, the paralysis of my eyes, arms, and legs has receded daily. After only a short period of time, I was able to urinate normally. My health improved so rapidly that I was soon able to return to my work part-time. Shortly after that, I was again examined at the Research Center and my reflexes were completely normal. The Budwig diet saved my life! Ten years later, I was given a thorough examination at the Center as a follow-up. My incredible recovery has been written up in many medical journals and I have become what they call a 'textbook case,' and all because of Dr. Johanna

Budwig, 's simple diet."

Timmy G.

Seven years ago Timmy G. was diagnosed as having Hodgkins disease. The child was operated on and underwent 24 radiation treatments, plus additional experimental therapies that the experts hoped would be of some small help.

When Timmy failed to respond favorably to these heroic measures, he was discharged as incurable, and given six months to live and sent home to die.

The desperate parents contacted specialists all over the world. A famous newspaper took up Timmy's cause and ran editorials pleading for someone to come forth who could offer hope for the life of a child. All the specialists who replied confirmed the cruel prognosis: There was no hope or help for Timmy.

At this dark hour the miracle the family had prayed for happened!

Timmy's mother told her story to the press: *"A friend sent me a printed piece about one of Dr. Budwig's speeches. This material gave us hope and I contacted Dr. Budwig.*

*In just **five days**, (on the Budwig regimen) Timmy's breathing became normal for the first time in almost two years.*

*From this day on, Timmy began to feel good again. He **went back to school**, started swimming and by winter he was doing craftwork. Everyone who knows him says how well he looks."*

At age 18 Timmy is showing great promise in his university work. He knows he owes his life to Dr. Budwig and thanks her daily in his prayers.

Whatever Happened to Dr. Budwig?

As for Dr. Budwig herself, she lived until 2003, when she passed away at 94. She had continued lecturing all over Europe through 1999. She had been nominated for **seven Nobel prizes** during her 50 plus years of advocacy about oils in the human body and treatment of cancer patients. Influential members of the allopathic medical community and the food (particularly margarine) processors always blocked her award of that deserved honor.

In Summary

Don't quibble. Don't put this off. Don't "wait to tell your doctor." In short, **just do it!!**

It's food. It costs nothing. It replaces one to two meals a day. It can't hurt you, unless the oil is rancid, which is pretty obvious. It'll smell. If it smells or tastes awful, don't use it. Take it back and get some fresh oil.

tricks Hormones

Lots of trivia on the chat board...high lignan oil vs. plain oil; ground flax seeds in addition to the oil or not; mix it by hand or in blender; flavor it with....well, you get the idea. **None of the people above worried about this stuff.** They just ate the mixture and got well.

Don't continue on your "normal" diet and expect to get well. This is a **lifetime commitment**. If you drop it after the 3-12 weeks it takes to heal you, you will be **very sorry**. Don't do that! Make it an everyday habit, as I have.

Antioxidants And The Budwig Diet

I frequently am asked why the folks at the Yahoo chat group (see above) insist that antioxidants are **not compatible** with the FO/CC mixture. Somewhere in her lectures, Dr. Budwig did state that supplements, including antioxidants, were unnecessary and might interfere with the effects of the FO/CC on the cells.

Despite what you may read at the Yahoo chat group, antioxidants are **not incompatible** with the FO/CC. As I discussed above, free radicals are a major source of damage to our cells. Mopping them up with antioxidants is just as necessary when using the FO/CC mixture. There is **absolutely no evidence** that the two are incompatible. What you will hear quoted is an opinion stated by Dr. Budwig that has no scientific basis. My regimen, as you will see, includes several items which act as effective antioxidants. These are necessary to our health and I take them every day, along with the FO/CC. Since 2000, hundreds of cancer patients have followed my regimen and are well now.

If you have any doubts about this, I suggest you look up the subject of "Antioxidants and Chemotherapy" on your favorite search engine. You will find that the same allegation – antioxidants interfere with chemo – has been made by oncologists for many years **despite hundreds of studies that prove this is not true**. In fact, if you insist on taking chemo, one of the best ways to offset the drastic side effects is to **take antioxidants**. But "the beat goes on" among the oncologists. "Be careful. These will interfere with your chemo." The statements at the FlaxseedOil2 chat group and other sources on this subject, in my opinion, reflect the **same ignoring of facts and adherence to an offhand statement by Dr. Budwig.**

Please, if you have any concern about this, just **separate by a couple of hours** your consumption of the FO/CC from the antioxidants in your regimen. Believe me, I do not find that necessary. I do my recommended regimen (see below) every day and I'm as close to "perfect health" as I could hope to be at my age.

Want to read some books? Caution: the first book with Dr. Budwig as the "author" is actually translations of her lectures from her German. To me, the book is virtually indecipherable. It is the typical rambling discourse of an extemperaneous lecture. Now, you are fairly warned.

"Flax Oil As a True Aid Against Arthritis, Heart Infarction, Cancer and Other Diseases," by Dr. Johanna Budwig, . Amazon price: $6.95.

"The Breuss Cancer Cure: Advice for the Prevention and Natural Treatment of Cancer, Leukemia and Other Seemingly Incurable Diseases," by Rudolf Breuss. Amazon price: $11.00.

"How To Fight Cancer and Win," by William L. Fischer. Amazon price: $19.95. Includes three chapters on Dr. Budwig's protocol.

"The Oil Protein Diet Cookbook," by Dr. Johanna Budwig. Amazon price: $10.36. Dr. Budwig gives you lots of great recipes to make her protocol "user-friendly."

Dr. Matthias Rath – Vitamin C & Lysine/Proline

The next treatment I would add to my cancer-fighting regimen is a mixture of Vitamin C, l-Lysine and l-Proline. The latter two are common amino acids. As I mentioned above in Chapter 1, this combination was discovered by Dr. Matthias Rath and Dr. Linus

Pauling in 1984. They later strengthened this compound by adding green tea extract, finding that it improved the effect by about 30%. They found that this combination **inhibited the process of metastasis of cancer cells**. You can study this concept in detail at Dr. Rath's web site: *http://www.drrathresearch.org/sci_discoveries/cancer.html*

If you have cancer, one of your first priorities is to **slow down or stop the process of metastasis** (spreading of cancer cells to other parts of the body). Metastasis and its effect on organs, blood, brain, bone marrow, etc. is what makes cancer more difficult to heal (not impossible).

There are several reasons I recommend this compound as a primary treatment. Like the first two treatments, this one is **gentle, non-toxic, and readily available.** Like the FO/CC, this one is also **inexpensive**. Not from Dr. Rath, but from **Our Health Co-op**. More on them in a minute. And finally, it gives you a "bonus" of **protection from or treatment of heart inflammation**.

None of the ingredients in Dr. Rath's formula are expensive. In fact, they are abundant and readily available. Nevertheless, his products (he has several) are all **quite expensive**. The reason is marketing. Like the drug companies, Dr. Rath spends a lot of money marketing his products.

With the effectiveness of this product for **both cancer and heart disease** and the publicity it has received for 24 years, there were bound to be **copycat products** developed. As I mentioned above, the only way to evaluate these products is the integrity of the source. Fortunately for you, there is a really inexpensive option competing with Dr. Rath's products ("Epican Forte," etc.).

Our Health Co-op, my favorite source for inexpensive (wholesale + 5%) natural products, sells something called **"Heart Plus."** The ingredients are Vitamin C, l-Lysine, l-Proline and Rose Hips. Except for the green tea extract, it is virtually identical to Dr. Rath's Epican Forte. Our Health Co-op sells the Green Tea Extract separately.

The Our Health Co-op price for Heart Plus is (drum roll, please) **$9.85**. Is that for one day? No, that's for 180 tablets (about a 30-day supply).

You can read about the theory behind Heart Plus and heart disease at:

http://www.OurHealthCoop.com/ourhealth_he.htm

Since heart disease is the number two killer and cancer is number one, this product gives you a **"double whammy."** It is much more effective than a cholesterol-lowering "statin" drug with none of the vast array of side effects, some fatal, from statin drugs.

This link will take you right to the ordering page for the Heart Plus:

http://store.ourhealthcoop.com/product_p/he.htm

To order their Green Tea Extract, you can go to:

http://store.ourhealthcoop.com/product_p/gt.htm

A one-month supply (90 veggie capsules) costs $9.58.

If I had cancer, I would take 6 of the Heart Plus (2-2-2) through the day and add three of the Green Tea Extract (1-1-1) at the same time. This will **slow down or completely stop** the spread of the cancer.

Notice that I devote **much less space** to Dr. Rath's compounds than to the FO/CC and immune system stimulants. Please don't interpret this as meaning they are less important. The only reason I can shorten the discourse is because Dr. Rath has such a wonderful web site, complete with **free PDF e-books and video tapes in four different languages**. Study his materials.

Greens and Enzymes

Bob Davis Whips Cancer

In November 2001, I discovered Bob Davis and his story. He has inspired me. But he has also furnished me with a ton of information about Complementary and Alternative Medicine (CAM) treatments for cancer. He will share them with you, too. Here, in his own words, is his story:

"I'm 88 years old, and I've overcome cancer twice!

In April 1996, I went to the hospital as an outpatient for an x-ray. They found that I had massive cancer. I had a mass in my abdomen a foot wide and several inches thick. Further, I had several masses in my chest, some of them 'the size of soft balls.' It was also determined that I had cancer in my bone marrow. I was immediately converted into an 'in' patient and started on a very heavy chemotherapy program. I had chemo in April, May, and June, with no effect on the cancer. It seemed to thrive on the stuff.

It was the middle of June when my doctor told me that the chemo wasn't working. He later told me that another treatment would kill me. I knew that this was true because my body was ravaged by the chemo. I was curled up in a fetal position unable to sleep or eat. I was emaciated and had excruciating pain all through my body.

I asked my doctor what we were going to do. He said, 'Try..........something else.'

The previous February I had called a college chum who had devastating arthritis. He couldn't climb stairs or drive his car. I asked him how he was doing and he said 'Fantastic!' He told me that he was taking an herbal product and it had eliminated his arthritis in three weeks. I asked him what it was and he said 'Dried green barley leaves.' He gave me the 800 number and I ordered a bottle for my wife who has arthritis.

It was the middle of June as I mention above, that I received a phone call from the owner of the company that provides the dried green barley pills [Florence Biros]. She asked me how I was doing on the pills. I told her that I wasn't using them. I had gotten them for my wife and they helped her when she remembered to take them.

I then said the most fortunate thing I have said in my life. I said, 'I'm fighting another battle.' She asked me what it was and I told her that it was cancer. She said, 'Oh, Mr. Davis, You don't know do you?' I asked her what was it that I didn't know and she said, 'Don't you know that cancer and arthritis can't grow in an alkaline body?' I told her that I had never heard that before. To make a long story short, I started taking the pills and in ten days my cancer was 95% gone! My next CT scan showed no cancer in my body and I have been cancer free ever since.

I was checked last month and I am still cancer free. I still take 20 200 mg. tablets of dried green barley every day. It costs me a whopping 85 cents or so.

112

Since then I have adopted a 95% (I do have birthday cake with a grandchild now and then) vegan diet that I really like. I feel better than I have in 40 years. People say I look younger. I have 'lotsa' energy.

I am eager to share information on cancer treatment and general health issues. I do occasionally speak at meetings on several related subjects. My favorite subject is ENZYMES!!!!

Bob Davis
Alternative Cancer Treatment Support
Feel free to contact me at ACTS@interhop.net"

Bob means it. If you want more information from him, he has it and will **share it with you.** He calls himself a reporter, not an adviser. Just send him an e-mail. He recently completed a web site. Check it out at:

http://www.cancer-success.com

He has been communicating with other cancer patients for nine years. He sent me copies of **40 e-mail messages** on a wide variety of CAM topics. Much of it was news to me. He has said I can share any of it I like with you. I am doing just that in this edition of my book.

Like another 88-year-old cancer survivor in my network, George Freaner, Bob is a **"nut" about enzymes**. Their enthusiasm has convinced this young buck (hey, I'm only 76!) to get up to speed on enzymes. I've read most of a telephone book-sized reference book called *"The Complete Book of Enzyme Therapy,"* by Dr. Anthony J. Cichoke. It is very interesting. Almost every malady you can think of can be traced to **one or another enzyme deficiency**. Do you remember what I said about cooked food above? That's right. **No enzymes.**

There are over 3,000 different types of enzymes in our bodies. Interestingly enough, the stuff that healed Bob Davis' cancer, green barley, contains all 3,000 of them, according to the discoverer, Dr. Yoshihide Hagiwara. Even before finishing the first few chapters of the Enzyme "encyclopedia," I had my whole family, including me, on the same thing Bob took. If you want to try it, it is called "Barley Power" and is put out by a company called Green Supreme, Inc. It comes in a **200 tablet bottle for $17.99**. Larger sizes are less per tablet. Order it at their website http://www.GreenSupreme.net or by calling (800) 358-0777 (they're in Pennsylvania) or (724) 946-9057 from outside the U.S. You'll be very glad you did.

Another Source

If you would like to try a different source, go to:

http://store.ourhealthcoop.com/product_p/gp.htm

Look over their product called **"Greens Plus."** Their 180 veggie capsules with a variety of "greens" and other ingredients, including barley, sell for $8.74.

Take Enough

Bob's experience points up one other very significant point. When you start on a therapy, **be sure you take enough** of it to have the effect you want. Bob takes 20 Barley Power tablets every day. No "half measures" for this lad (hey, he feels like a young stud of 40!).

By the way, Bob Davis has no financial connection with Green Supreme, Inc. (or any other products). They are currently a **sponsor of my web talk radio show** and thereby help me to pay the overhead. I don't make any profit from that show. When I accept a sponsor like Green Supreme, it's because I believe in **their product and their integrity.**

The Importance of pH

Remember Florence Biros. She's the Green Supreme company owner. In Bob Davis' account of his treatment, she's the one who said *"Don't you know that cancer and arthritis **cannot grow in an alkaline body?"*** What exactly did she mean by that?

Your body fluids vary somewhat throughout your day in the degree to which they are alkaline or acid [except your blood, which your body keeps within a narrow range by whatever means necessary]. The easiest way to determine whether your body is in an alkaline or acid state is to **test your saliva**.

At the same "800" number above I gave you for the "Barley Power," you can order a roll or two of **pH test strips**. An 8-foot roll costs about $9.50. Every morning when you first wake up (before you eat or drink anything) you can put a **two-inch strip** under your tongue for a couple of seconds and it will show you where you are on the alkaline to acid scale. Ideal is around 6.4. This is what is called your "alkaline stores." To confirm the science behind this, please see a very informative web site:

http://biomedx.com/pH/page5.html

With our typical acid diet, most of you with cancer will find that your pH is 5.5 or less. If the Barley Power or similar enzyme booster and alkalinity products are working correctly, this should **correct in 2-3 weeks to the 6.4 level** and stay there as long as you continue to take the "Greens" tablets, capsules or powder.

If you'd like a lot more background and detail on this subject, you will find it in the book *"The pH Miracle: Balance Your Diet,*

Reclaim Your Health" by Dr. Robert O. Young. A check of Amazon.com showed this book available for as little as $3.63. As one reviewer says: *"I feel Dr. Young is going after the underlying 'cause' of disease and not just traditionally treating an ill with a pill!"*

A Cancer-Fighting Diet

Next in order of importance for you, the cancer patient is a **radically different diet**. It is almost certain that if your diet had been perfect, you wouldn't have cancer. None of us eat the perfect diet. **But now, you must!** No kidding.

Nutritionists

I have read at least 15 books by nutritionists and corresponded with several of them. My conclusion, after eight years of searching, is that all nutritionist advice is ------ **opinion** (with two exceptions). Yep, that's right. There is very little science here. There is lots of disagreement. What is acid for one person is alkaline for another, and so on. It fosters a lot of confusion among those of us trying to reform our diets.

Atkins Diet, Eat Right 4 Your Type, South Beach Diet, Patrick Quillin's "Beating Cancer With Nutrition," Jordan Rubin's "The Maker's Diet," Mike Anderson's "The RAVE Diet & Lifestyle," Donna Gates' "The Body Ecology Diet," Diana Dyer's "A Dietician's Cancer Story," "The Stockholm Protocol," Dr. Flavin-Koenig's "Foods to Avoid" and "Foods to Eat" lists for cancer patients (which I have published in earlier versions of this book) --- **ALL are opinions**. I find statements in each of them that I disagree with or challenge with "Where's the science behind that opinion?"

What are my "two exceptions?" One is *"The China Study"* by T. Colin Campbell, Ph.D. This book is science. Peer-reviewed, carefully documented science. Please don't waste your money on other diet books. This one will tell you all you need to know – except one thing. What about food allergies?

Fotunately for us, the world's "living expert" on food allergies, Dr. Keith Scott-Mumby has collected his 30 years of experience in a book called *"Diet Wise."* Every one of us, according to Dr. Scott-Mumby, has at least one food allergy. This is the main reason why standard diets don't work for everyone. Please get his book at http://www.DietWiseBook.com and read it. You will be amazed.

There is more information on this subject and both these books in my Booklet #1 *"Stop Your Aging With Diet"* which is at the end of this book (under the same cover).

So, having trashed almost all the "expert" nutritionists, what do I recommend? Well, I'll tell you. It's quite simple. There are just **five (5) "no-noes."** Once you have determined your food allergies, if you can avoid putting any of these five things in your mouth, you will be fighting your cancer as effectively as possible. Except for these five, you can eat **as much and as often as you like.**

The Five No-Noes

Any theory has to start with assumptions. Before I list my five "no-noes," I have to assume you are not doing any of the following: smoking or chewing **tobacco**; drinking **sodas** (diet or otherwise); taking **recreational drugs**; drinking anything with **alcohol** in it; drinking **caffiene** (except maybe one cup of coffee a day).

OK, you're not doing anything stupid. Then, all you have to do is avoid the following:

1. **Sugar – in any form**. (Stevia, Agave nectar or xylitol are the only sweeteners I recommend for cancer patients). This is a **lifetime commitment**, not only during your recovery.

2. **Processed food – in any form**. The simplest way I can explain this is "If it is not in the form God made it, you don't eat it." Again, this is a **lifetime commitment.** Processed food is the cause of most major illness. Does this make it difficult to go out to eat – at friends and relatives houses or in a restaurant? You bet. "Is he saying I need to take my food with me?" **You bet!**

3. **Animal protein**. Not just red meat, but ALL animal protein. Fish, chicken, seafood, shellfish, eggs. It is all very difficult for your body to digest. You are taking 40% of your body's energy away from fighting the cancer to digest your food. This is not the way to get well. This one can be relaxed when you are "cancer-free" (see below). But only a little. One piece of chicken or fish a week, for example. Don't believe me? Please read *"The China Study."*

4. **Dairy**. Milk, ice cream, cheese, butter. Again, all very hard for your body to digest. Any human over five years of age has no lactase in their body. Lactase is the enzyme necessary to digest dairy products. Even if the milk comes from the cow next door, don't drink it. Many laboratory studies show that **dairy promotes cancer.** What about the cottage cheese? Remember, I said it **loses all its dairy properties** when you mix it with the flaxseed oil. Dozens of people I have worked with who are "lactose intolerant" are eating the FO/CC mixture every day with no problems.

5. **Gluten**. Bread, cereal, pasta. 30% of adults are allergic to gluten. Most of them don't know it because the allergic reaction is frequently delayed for hours or days. The main problem with this category of food, however, is its **high "glycemic index."** It turns into glucose rapidly. If you want to feed your cancer cells, eat gluten. Otherwise, avoid it. Most health food stores these days have "gluten-free" crackers and sprouted bread-like products.

   [There is a handy "acronym" to help you avoid grains with gluten. It is **"BROWS."** The "B" is for barley (grain, not the young barley leaf in the Barley Power pills); "R" is for rye; "O" is for oats; "W" is for wheat; and "S" is for spelt. Avoid them all.]

What's Left?

Every time I go over this list of "no-noes" with a cancer patient on the phone, I get the same response – **"What's left for me to eat?"** Actually, there are lots of things. You just need to look around in places you may not have looked before.

Let's see what is left:

1. **Raw, whole vegetables**. The easiest way to cleanse your entire digestive system and get all the nutrients and fiber you need is to eat **large salads** with a wide variety of raw veggies and a little olive oil and lemon juice on the top (no other salad dressing). What veggies? Dark, green leafy stuff (kale, kohlrabi, spinach, etc.); broccoli; cauliflower; cucumbers; onions (red and yellow); bell peppers (red, yellow and green); radishes; tomatoes; squash; carrots; leeks; lentils; sprouts of all kinds; and on and on. Buy "organic" veggies, if you can afford them. Just realize that this label is not controlled by anybody. There is no

guarantee that veggies so labeled were perfectly grown, harvested and shipped locally. Potatoes and rice are high on the glycemic index. Steam some vegetables – asparagus, green beans, brussel sprouts, etc. – that cannot be eaten raw.

2. **Sprouted breads** of all kinds – english muffins, etc. Just look around the health food store. You'll find lots of "gluten-free" products.

3. **Preservative-free bread** – "Ezekiel" and "Genesis" brands and similar have recently introduced "gluten free" options. You'll find them in the frozen food section of your health food store. They have to be kept in the freezer because they have no chemical preservatives added to make you sick. We toast this bread and enjoy it with a little olive oil (no butter, remember?) all the time.

4. **Cereals** made with millet, quinoa, amaranth, buckwheat, etc. and no gluten. Use almond milk on them, not soy milk. (Soy is VERY controversial. Why eat anything so controversial when you're sick? Let others prove who's right.) Just be careful that neither the cereal nor the milk has any artificial or real sweeteners and preservatives.

5. **Fruit.** Except for the berries or pineapple (another good cancer-fighting fruit) you put in the FO/CC smoothie in the morning, try to limit your fruit to one piece of whole fruit (apple, banana, handful of grapes, etc.) a day. No fruit juice. It blasts your pancreas with fruit sugar.

What about **vegetable juice?** I recommend you **avoid it**. Not because it is unhealthy. It steals your appetite from the foods above – all of which have, along with other nutrients – **FIBER**. All cancer patients need to eat a lot of fiber (35 grams per day or more). You cannot afford to be constipated.

There is a small minority of people who just do not "thrive" on a pure "vegan" diet like that described above. I urge you to at least try the above approach for a couple of weeks. If you really feel weak, add some good organic chicken or some cold water fish (salmon, tuna, etc.) and see if it helps. Try to keep it to **once or twice a week.**

It's not obvious, but the above method of eating acts as a very efficient and thorough **cleanse of your entire digestive system**.

DoctorYourself.com

Another interesting article on nutrition and cancer, especially the importance of vitamins and treatment with Vitamin C, is at:

http://www.DoctorYourself.com/cancer_2.html

Diet Trumps DNA As The Cause of Cancer

Here's a short article from one of my recent (July, 2008) newsletters. I encourage you to read the article I refer to at Dr. Jon Barron's web site. He is a font of information whom I trust.

"Well, finally, there is a study which, as sort of an accidental finding, has determined that diet is the key. This was a recent study of men with prostate cancer. It found that diet and lifestyle changes could 'switch off' some 453 cancer-promoting genes, while simultaneously 'switching on' some 48 cancer- fighting genes. Does this study prove that diet and lifestyle trump DNA? You decide. Dr. Jon Barron is a holistic physician whom I admire. I suggest that you read his comments on this study at this website:

www.JonBarron.org/newsletters/07-07-2008.php"

Summary On The Cancer-Fighting Diet

I read about cancer every day. I've counselled hundreds (thousands?) of cancer patients on the phone and by e-mail. There is no doubt. What we put in our mouths, more than any other one thing, is a very common **cause** of any original cancer episode and of **recurrence**.

We've talked a lot in these pages about supplements and we'll soon discuss enzyme therapy. Certainly, many of these substances can contribute to your recovery. However, the **best and cheapest** way to restore your body's metabolism to its natural balanced state and regain your health is to **eat right.**

Do you realize?

- o The average American consumes **170 pounds of sugar per year!** Don't believe it? Just take a look at your pantry. All that sucrose, corn syrup, caramel color and fructose is just sugar in disguise.

- o **Acrylamide**, a proven carcinogen (cancer causing agent), is only allowed in your drinking water at a level of **0.12 micrograms per serving** by the Environmental Protection Agency (EPA). McDonald's French Fries, large, 6 oz. serving, contain **72 micrograms or 600 times the EPA limit**. Burger King, Wendy's, KFC, etc. are just slightly lower. Still want that "super size?"

- o The **processed food** we eat has had virtually all the good nutrients, plus all the digestive enzymes, processed out of it. Our bodies **can't produce the enzymes** needed to digest this stuff. Do you really think the food manufacturers are concerned about your health? Guess again, my friend.

- o The Standard American Diet (SAD) is **highly acidic**. In a 300-page book called *"The pH Miracle,"* (see above) Dr. Robert Young, a microbiologist and nutritionist argues convincingly that the **most important marker** of good health is the pH level.

.....and there's lots more evidence that we **eat** ourselves into degenerative conditions of all kinds.

Vitamin/Mineral Supplement

The sixth item of the "Bill Henderson Protocol" (i.e. **"What I would do if I were you."**) is Dr. Williams' Daily Advantage vitamin/mineral supplement. I described this in Chapter 3, including a list of all 69 ingredients. Please review this now. It is essential to "fill all the holes" in any diet – including the one we described above.

This supplement comes in plastic packets, each of which contains 8 capsules. I have taken two of these packets (the normal dose) every **day for the past 12 years** or so. I attribute my perfect health at age 76 to this product. If you wonder why I recommend it, that's why. It works for me and I believe it will for you. If you find something better, by all means buy it and let me know what it is.

Summary of the Self-Treatments

Before we go any farther, let's summarize this six-part **"protocol."** Ideally, I'd like this summary to be on your refrigerator as a daily reminder of the essential steps I would do (and I hope you will) to **overcome cancer.** Here they are:

1. **Immune System Stimulation** – Transfer Point Beta-1,3D Glucan. One 500mg capsule per 50 pounds (23 kilos) of body weight daily – in the morning, 30 minutes before eating or drinking anything. Source: http://www.AboutBetaGlucan.com/bspecial or call Phyllis or Michael at (800) 746-7640 or (678) 560-1808 (Eastern time).

2. **Cottage Cheese/Flaxseed Oil "Smoothie."** Six tablespoons of flaxseed oil mixed by hand or with a single-blade hand mixer with about 2/3 cup of organic, 1% fat cottage cheese. Add berries and nuts and a little stevia in the blender. Adjust the mixture to your taste. Blend on "Liqueify" setting. Eat it as soon as it is blended. Order flaxseed oil from Barleans at (800) 445-3529 (Pacific time).

3. **Heart Plus and Green Tea Extract**. Six capsules of Heart Plus (2-2-2) and three caplets (1-1-1) of the Green Tea Extract. They should be taken together with food or between meals. It doesn't matter. Source for both: http://www.ourhealthcoop.com

4. **Barley Power.** Twenty tablets per day. Take 6 or 7 about 15 minutes before each meal. If you are not eating three meals a day, take them two hours after eating. Source: Green Supreme, Inc. (800) 358-0777 or (724) 946-9057 (Eastern time) or http://www.GreenSupreme.net.

5. **Cancer-fighting diet**. Avoid foods on the five "no-noes" list [sugar; processed food; animal protein; dairy; and gluten]. Maximize the raw, whole vegetables. For variety,

eat gluten-free, sprouted bread products, flaxseed crackers, cereals (millet, quinoa, etc. without gluten and with unsweetened almond milk), lentils, seeds and nuts (no peanuts).

6. **Vitamin/Mineral Supplement**. Take two packets of Daily Advantage daily. Source: Mountain Home Nutritionals (800) 888-1415 (Eastern time) or http://www.DrDavidWilliams.com

That's all, folks. If you follow this regimen **diligently (every day)** for about 6-8 weeks, you will not just improve your condition; you will **probably be "cancer-free."** If not, there are literally 300 plus other gentle, non-toxic cancer treatments to try. We'll cover some of them in the following pages.

Maintenance Doses

What about when you're cancer-free? What then? Good question. You've gotten back an HCG Urine Test (see below) in the 40's and completed your celebration. What should you do now? Here are some suggestions based on what I do myself every day for prevention:

1. **Immune System Stimulation**. I would continue taking the Beta 1-3D Glucan daily but at the one capsule level, once a day. When I feel some form of virus or other infection coming on, I immediately up the dose to the "therapeutic" dose (see above) for just a couple of days.

2. **Cottage Cheese/Flaxseed Oil "Smoothie."** I would continue eating this but just cut the dose about in half. That's what my wife and I do every morning. I would never miss a dose of this wonderful elixir. If you want to ensure

your cancer will not recur, please take this advice seriously.

3. **Heart Plus and Green Tea Extract.** I would eliminate this combination but keep any supply you have handy in case you have a recurrence of the cancer.

4. **Barley Power.** I would cut back to 7 or 8 of these pills a day, but continue taking them at the rate of 3 or 4 before each meal.

5. **Cancer-Fighting Food.** I would relax this set of eating habits (it's not a "diet") but only slightly. For example, I would continue to avoid sugar in any form and processed food in any form. I would add a little animal protein (fish, chicken, eggs) to my diet about twice a week. I would continue to avoid the dairy and gluten products along with meat (beef, pork, etc.).

6. **Vitamin/Mineral Supplement.** I would continue to take the Daily Advantage at the same dose (2 packets of capsules per day).

Features of This Protocol

Before we explore other treatments, let me point out some of the features of this regimen which may not be obvious:

It addresses the **four characteristics** of all cancer, not just the symptoms. Those characteristics are: **Lack of oxygen uptake by the cells**; **excess acidity; excess toxins; and a weak immune system.**

The **"die-off"** of the cancer cells is **gentle** and occurs over a 2-3 week period. Usually, the effects of this are quite bearable.

However, there always are some detoxification effects – pain in the liver/kidney area, unusual bowel movements and urine, rashes, mild nausea, fever, etc. All of these are quite normal. Medication you take for these symptoms slow down the healing process.

Frequently, the cancer "markers" (particularly blood tests like the CEA, CA-125, etc.) will show a **"spike"** in the count. This could last for several weeks. This is normal and is caused by the increase in "antigens" in your blood from the dying cancer cells. Frequently, this will cause unnecessary panic, especially if you are still listening to your oncologist. He/she will want to begin chemotherapy or some other drastic treatment. **Relax** and wait a few days.

This is a **very inexpensive** regimen. For the first 6-8 weeks, while taking the immune system stimulant at the therapeutic dose, the cost is about $155 (U.S. dollars) per month. Of course, in countries outside the U.S., it will be somewhat more because of the shipping costs from the U.S. sources. After you are "cancer-free" the cost to continue the regimen at the maintenance level is about **$104 per month**.

These products are mostly available **anywhere in the world.** For example, Our Health Co-op (Heart Plus and Green Tea Extract) will ship to any country with a choice of shipping options. Green Supreme, Inc. (Barley Power) will do likewise. Flaxseed oil and organic cottage cheese (also called "quark") are available in the health food stores in most countries. Better Way Health will ship the Transfer Point Beta Glucan anywhere. Dr. Williams' Daily Advantage can only be ordered online for shipment in the U.S. or to APO/FPO (military) addresses. You will need to substitute another vitamin/mineral supplement in countries outside the U.S.

If the cancer patient insists on following the chemo/radiation recommendations of the cancer doctors, this regimen will **offset most of the side effects**.

I have developed this "protocol" over the last six years, primarily with **feedback from cancer patients about what works.**

Causes of Cancer That Are First Priority

There are two causes of cancer which are quite common and which will preclude the above regimen (or any other regimen) from working until they are addressed.

Emotional Trauma & Stress

Dr. Ryke Geerd Hamer has spent quite a bit of time in jail in the last several years. Why? He has discovered what he thinks is the key to all cancers and most other degenerative conditions. As you know by now, this type of opinion spooks Big Pharma into **full attack mode**.

Dr. Hamer developed testicular cancer himself in 1978. It appeared a few months after his son was shot to death in Italy. He began to investigate the connection. Here is a web site with an enormous amount of information on Dr. Hamer's theory:

http://www.GermanNewMedicine.ca

Dr. Hamer is a medical doctor. What he discovered after investigating **40,000 cases (of which about 12,000 were cancer cases)** is that a particular area of the brain is associated with each organ of the body. Emotional trauma, he says, always affects an organ's function. Each cancer, he found, was connected with a particular **emotional trauma**. He has labeled his theories "German New Medicine" (the term "New Medicine" was already taken).

Needless to say, the medical "establishment" did not welcome Dr. Hamer's findings. In fact, he has been **repeatedly persecuted and jailed** in Germany and France over the last several years.

From my experience, I agree with him that many **(not all)** cancers develop from emotional trauma and the stress that follows it. This stress can also be long-term – e.g. running a business, living in a difficult relationship, caring for an aging relative, etc.

If you are experiencing this kind of stress now, you must address it and resolve it before you can recover from cancer. One of the great forms of treatment is called Emotional Freedom Technique (EFT). You can begin researching this, including a list of practitioners, at Gary Craig, the inventor's, web site:

http://www.emofree.com

I also suggest you read Dr. Brad Nelson's book *"The Emotion Code."* It is available at Amazon.com. It's an effective method of freeing your mind and body of **"trapped emotions."** It is something I would try before seeking out an EFT practitioner. Dr. Nelson's approach is strictly self-help. My wife and I have tried it and **it works.**

Check out Dr. Nelson's web sites:

http://www.TheEmotionCode.com

…and

http://www.DrBradleyNelson.com

Root Canal Teeth

At least **60% of the cancer patients** I deal with have root canal-filled teeth (some as many as 10 or 11). There is no question that these teeth cause cancer and many other degenerative conditions. If you have any root canal-filled teeth, you must have them removed **immediately** by a "biological dentist" if you want to recover from your cancer.

What is a "biological dentist?" Well, the simplest description is that he/she is a dentist who is **more concerned with your health than your smile**. Another distinguishing characteristic is that he/she will not do root canal fillings and will urge you to have any in your mouth removed as soon as possible.

Please don't take my word for this. Read the best book on the subject I know of, because of who wrote it. The book is *"Root Canal Cover-Up."* The author is George Meinig, D.D.S, F.A.C.D. Those letters mean "Doctor of Dental Surgery," and "Fellow of the American College of Dentistry." He was a **very prominent dentist.** (He passed away in 2008 at 91).

Dr. Meinig began doing root canal fillings on his patients' teeth in 1943. In 1948, he was one of the 19 **founders of the American Association of Endodontists** (root canal therapists). When he retired in 1993, he was honored, along with the other three surviving founders at the 50th anniversary celebration of the AAE.

In 1993, shortly after his retirement, Dr. Meinig learned of the 1,174 pages of research done on root canal teeth by **Dr. Weston Price**, D.D.S., F.A.C.D. and 60 fellow research dentists. Their findings had been **suppressed by the American Dental Association since 1925.** This research, done over 20 years, showed, beyond any doubt, that there was no safe way to do a root canal filling. Not only that, but the research established root canal teeth as the **cause** of many serious degenerative conditions, including cancers.

The Paracelsus Clinic in Switzerland has treated cancer patients **since 1958**. A part of this clinic is a Biological Dentist Section. Every cancer patient who comes to the clinic has his/her mouth **cleaned of root canal-filled teeth before any other cancer treatment is done**. In 2004, the clinic's Director, Dr. Thomas Rau, feeling that most breast cancer patients they were treating had root canal teeth, decided to do a study. He reviewed the records of the last 150 of their breast cancer patients. He found that **147 of them (98%)** had one or more root canal teeth on the **same meridian** as their original breast cancer tumor. He believes there is no doubt that this was the primary cause of their cancers.

Please, if you have any root canal teeth, treat removing them from your mouth as **your number one priority**. You will not get well until you do this. Once it is done properly, you may **need very little other treatment to get well.**

Finding one of the biological dentists who can remove the tooth/teeth **properly** may not be easy. As of 2008, one of the best ways to locate one of these people is to call the office of Dr. Hal Huggins in Colorado Springs, Colorado (Mountain Time). Dr. Huggins and Dr. Thomas Levy, an M.D., worked together on a study of root canal-filled teeth for six years – from 1994 to 2000. Dr. Levy told me that they had removed 5,000 root canal-filled teeth. He said each tooth they removed was tested n the lab. **Every one of them had toxins coming out of it that were "more toxic than botulism"** (Dr. Levy's words).

To get a referral to a biological dentist near you from the directory which Dr. Huggins and Dr. Levy put together, call (866) 948-4638 (Mountain Time). **Warning:** Do not discuss your condition with the person who answers the phone unless you want a "sales pitch" on Dr. Huggins' healing regimen.

What We Put In Our Mouth

After eight years of talking to cancer patients on the phone about the cause of their cancers, I'm convinced that if the two causes above don't explain why you got cancer, the only remaining cause is **what we put in our mouth**. We talked about the high percentage of cancers among smokers above. Lots of cancers are caused by smoking. But **many more are caused by our food**. Smoking has decreased dramatically in the U.S. in the last 50 years. But the rate of cancer has risen dramatically. Why? It's the food we eat.

Cooked food has **no enzymes and few nutrients**. Yet, our culture has evolved a worship of chefs and cooked food. Believe me, eating cooked food is at least part of the **cause of most cancers**.

The food we buy in the supermarket has been processed to the point that no sensible animal would eat it. Rats in laboratories have been fed **MSG** (monosodium glutamate) and **made obese**. The only difference in their diet was the MSG added. There are literally **30 different names for MSG** – carrageenan, hydrolyzed vegetable protein, natural flavors, etc., etc. There is no question that it is the **major cause of obesity in this country**. Just read the labels. If you can find one processed food without some form of MSG in it, you get the prize.

High fructose corn syrup is in the majority of the food you eat. It is many times as harmful to your body as refined sugar, which is bad enough. Yet, after MSG, it is the **most common additive in our food**. It is addictive. Your children get hooked on certain breakfast cereals. Why? The high fructose corn syrup in them.

And don't get me started on **chemicals, artificial coloring** and all the other additives in processed food. Face it, folks. The food manufacturers are **not concerned about your health.** They are concerned with appearance, shelf life and taste. Only **you** are concerned about your health. And unless you believe the above few paragraphs, your food is going to make you sick.

Here are two quotes for you to think about:

1958: "According to present government statistics, **one of every six persons** in the population will die of cancer. It will not be long before the entire population will have to decide whether we will all die of cancer or change fundamentally all our living and **nutritional conditions**." (Max Gerson, author of *"A Cancer Therapy."*)

2002: "Today, **one of every two men and one of every three women** in the United States alone will **confront cancer** over the course of their lives." (Andrew von Eschenbach, M.D., Director of the National Cancer Institute in *"Everyone's Guide to Cancer Therapy"*)

What to do? See the "five no-noes" I list above. If you want to **prevent cancer**, just **eliminate** those five types of food from your diet. You also might want to start eating some flaxseed oil and cottage cheese for breakfast – as I do every morning. Keep your immune system strong with an **immune boosting product** (Transfer Point Beta Glucan is a good choice). Take some **Barley Power pills** every day (see above). Take a daily vitamin/mineral product like Daily Advantage. These **habits,** along with some daily exercise and sunshine, have **kept me healthy**. They will do the same for you.

How Do I Know My Regimen Is Working?

One of the most frequent questions I get when I counsel cancer patients is this one. Is there a test that will tell me **conclusively** that I'm overcoming the cancer? Well, yes there is. Only one that I know of. But it is a good one, proven over 70 years as the most **accurate** way to determine the level of "abnormally dividing cells" in your body.

These cells occur only if: a) You are pregnant; b) You have a huge wound which is healing; or c) You have cancer. Most cancer tests (CT/PET scans, MRI's, blood tests, etc.) are **ambiguous**. In short, they do not tell you conclusively whether you're getting better – overcoming the cancer. The reports on the tests contain language that is obtuse and incomprehensible to the patient. **This test is different.**

It is called the **HCG Urine Cancer Test**. HCG stands for *Human Chorionic Gonadotropin*. Knowing that name is not important. However, you may have heard of it in connection with the pregnancy test. That test gives a "Yes/No" answer.

This test looks at the same phenomenom (abnormally dividing cells) but it tells you the **relative number or level of these cells regardless of where they are in your body or where they started.** Doesn't this sound like a useful fact to know?

The test returns a single number. If that number is 50 or more, you have cancer that requires treatment. If it is **zero to 49**, you have the normal number of "abnormally dividing cells" (cancer cells) in **everyone's body every da**y.

The beauty of this test is that it provides you with an **accurate trend.** After you get the second of these tests, if the second number is lower, you can be sure that **what you are doing is working**. Hopefully, this result will inspire you to continue until you are "cancer-free" (in the zero to 49 range).

The cost for the test is $50 US Dollars. No doctor's prescription is required. Compare this to the AMAS blood test (covered earlier in this book) which costs $135 plus shipping and requires a doctor's prescription. Also, the urine test is **more accurate** than the AMAS test.

You send the $50 to a U.S. address and then include a Xerox copy of the money order or cashier's check in the package you send to the Navarro Clinic in Manila in The Philippines. Priority Mail takes about 5-6 days to get there and costs about $6.50. You will usually get the results back in about 8 days IF you send them your e-mail address along with the dry urine sediment sample. If you use regular mail, it takes anywhere from 6 weeks to forever. Fed Ex costs over $47.

The following procedure is not hard. I've done it a couple of times. The last number I got was 42.5. I have left the description verbatim as I received it for those of you who insist on scientific evidence.

Why Get An HCG Urine Cancer Test?

Developed in the late 1930's by the renowned oncologist, the late Dr. Manuel D. Navarro, the test detects the presence of HCG in urine. It indicates the presence of cancer cells even before signs or symptoms develop. Dr. Navarro found HCG to be elevated in all types of cancers.

The test is based on a theory proposed by Dr. Howard Beard and other researchers who contend that cancer is related to a

misplaced trophoblast cell that becomes malignant in a manner similar to pregnancy in that they both secrete HCG. As a consequence, a measure of the amount of HCG found in the blood or urine is also a measure of the **degree of malignancy**. The higher the number, the greater the severity of the cancer.

[**Comment:** Over the last six years or so, I have heard from **hundreds** of people who have taken this test. Most of their first numbers come back between 53 and 63. The theoretical range of numbers from this test is zero to 10,000. Dr. Efren Navarro, the son of the inventor of this test who currently runs the Navarro Clinic in the Philippines, says he has seen some **"over 1,000."** The highest I've heard of is 103.

The test is **quite accurate.** A drop in the number on the second test of even one or two points is a very accurate indication that **"what you are doing is working."** The message you get back from the Navarro Clinic will say something like "+4 [54.3 I.U.] This number indicates.....etc." The "+4" actually means "plus or minus 4." It's an indication of the lab's opinion of the accuracy of the number. In my experience, the number is much more accurate than that. Once your number from this test is 49 or below, you can schedule your **"Cancer-Free" party**.]

Urine, as opposed to blood or serum, is the preferred specimen for the test. In 1980, Papapetrou and co-authors reported the correctness of the urine specimen to be used in HCG test. In 32 proven cancer cases, the urine test gave **31 positive results** while only **12 positive results were reported using blood**.

[Many people ask me "Why send it to the Philippines? Aren't there labs in the U.S. which can do this test?" Unfortunately, the answer is no. Labs in the U.S. do only the blood version of this test. It is **much less trouble** for the lab workers, but, as you can see above, the urine test is much more accurate.]

HCG has been found to undergo glycosylation in the liver as it travels in circulating blood. Thus, the HCG molecule cannot be detected. The molecule does not undergo this process in the kidney and therefore the molecule **remains intact in the urine.**

The test detects the presence of brain cancer as early as **29 months before symptoms appear;** 27 months for fibrosarcoma of the abdomen; 24 months for skin cancer; 12 months for cancer of the bones.

Currently, many cancer patients take advantage of the **diagnostic accuracy** of this test as an indicator of the **effectiveness of their specific mode of therapy**. Patients follow a simple direction for preparing a dry extract from the urine sample. The powdery extract is mailed to the Navarro Medical Clinic in Manila, The Philippines, where the HCG testing is performed.

How to Prepare The Sample

(1) From an early morning urine, take 50 cc (1.7 oz.) and add 200 cc (7 oz.) of acetone (can be purchased from hardware store or pharmacy) and 5 cc (.2 oz) of alcohol, either rubbing or ethyl. Stir and mix well.

(2) Let it stand in the refrigerator for 4-6 hours until sediment is formed. Throw off about half of the urine-acetone mixture without losing any sediment. [Make sure the sediment stays at the bottom of the container -- i. e. don't stir it up.] Filter the remainder through a coffee filter or laboratory filter paper.

(3) When filtration is over, dry the filter with its sediment. Fold and wrap in aluminum foil. Send by Priority Mail to the Navarro Medical Clinic (address below) including a Xerox copy of the money order or cashier's check with the patient's name, address, sex, and age and a brief clinical history and/or diagnosis. Also, **be SURE to include your e-mail address.** This will speed up your receipt of the results by at least 4-6 weeks.

(4) PRECAUTION: No sexual contact for 12 days for female patients before collecting the urine sample. For males, no sexual contact for 18-24 hours before collecting the urine sample. DO NOT SEND URINE IF THE PATIENT IS PREGNANT.

Send the above information and the sample to:

Navarro Medical Clinic
Dr. Efren Navarro
3553 Sining Street
Morningside Terrace
Santa Mesa, Manila 1016
Philippines

The Navarro Clinic phone number from the U.S. is: 011-(632) 714-7442

At the same time, send a money order or cashier's check (no personal checks, please) for $50 to:

Mrs. Erlinda Suarez
631 Peregrine Drive
Palatine, Illinois 60067-7005 USA

Mrs. Suarez is related to Dr. Navarro. Her phone number is: (847) 359-3634 . [Evening calls appreciated]. Normally, there is no need to call her. Just send her the $50.

Background – "The HCG Immunity Link" by Ruth Sackman

Here is the background on the nature of this test as written by Ruth Sackman. Ruth is 93 as this book is written. She and her late husband have helped cancer patients recover for over 35 years. She is a truly remarkable lady.

"Dr. Howard Beard, a biochemist and cancer patient, found that he could monitor his cancer by doing the human chorionic

138

gonadotrophin (HCG) immunoassay to determine how actively his body was producing unnecessary cells or controlling cell production at a normal level. This HCG test is used to determine pregnancy, a natural process, whereby the body is producing excess cells for the development of a fetus.

Dr. Beard's theory was that if HCG levels rose but no fetus was developing, then abnormal cell production was taking place which, to him, signified a cancer problem. Dr. Manuel Navarro agreed with this philosophy and established a measurement to diagnose cancer. A tumor would not be clinically evident immediately but in time might manifest in men as well as women.

Two scientists with the West London Hospital, Helen Davies and S. F. Contractor were interested in one of the most mysterious biological processes – how the body knew when birth was ready at the end of nine months gestation. They reported in the British journal Nature that they believe birth is really a process of rejection initiated by the body's own defense system.

The reason this rejection is controlled is because above normal amounts of HCG appear in the mother's urine during pregnancy. HCG, they believe, prevents the mother's sentry cells (lymphocytes) from recognizing the foreign protein (fetus). The HCG levels remain high until just before birth when a drop in HCG triggers the rejection of the fetus and birth occurs. Without such recognition, rejection cannot take effect. Ergo, when the HCG titre is above normal [above 49] on the HCG test, cancer cell rejection does not take place.

Therefore, Dr. Beard's theory of measuring HCG levels has a sound scientific basis. Low levels of HCG allow the body to reject abnormal protein just as it rejects the fetus and high levels interfere with the body's ability to build the lymphocytes necessary to effect rejection of cancer cells.

This theory validates Dr. Beard's conclusion that the HCG measurement found in the urine was a competent system to diagnose and monitor cancer cell activity."

Bottom line: I recommend you get an HCG Urine Test from Dr. Navarro's Clinic **as soon as possible after your cancer diagnosis**. This will give you a "baseline" number. If I were the cancer patient, this is **the only test I would need.** I would avoid CT/PET scans for two reasons: the preparation for that test requires me to **drink glucose to "light up"** the cancer cells [does this sound healthy to you?]; and then the test itself exposes me to the equivalent of about 20-30 chest x-rays. All forms of radiation are cumulative in your body. Radiation is a **proven carcinogen (cancer-causing agent)**. MRI's are magnetic energy, not radiation. Still, they are very expensive and quite ambiguous. Cancer marker blood tests (CEA, CA-125, etc.) would be unnecessary if I were doing the Navarro Urine Cancer Test. They are less accurate.

How Often Should This Test Be Repeated?

Dr. Navarro says the optimum time between tests is 8 weeks. My guess is that you will get impatient and want to see that next number in less than 8 weeks. I'd wait at least 6-7 weeks between tests.

Other Effective Cancer Therapies

In this next section, I will describe several other treatments I have researched. All of these are valid and have worked for many people. However, I suggest you try the regimen outlined above for 6-8 weeks [and measure your success with at least two Navarro Urine Cancer Tests] **before you begin adding other treatments.** In most cases I have dealt with, they are unnecessary.

There are two reasons I suggest this: First, too great a variety of treatments will risk your **losing patience** with the whole regimen and abandoning it too soon – "This is too complex – I give up!" Above all, I don't want this to happen to you; and, second, the above regimen has worked now for so many people **with all types and stages of cancer** – all over the world – that I want you to give it a fair trial.

Remember, full, **100% commitment** to almost any well designed regimen will almost guarantee its success – the old **"mind-body effect."** The best chance you have of beating cancer is to make **"drastic" and "permanent"** changes to your lifestyle.

Of course, you, and only you, are in charge of your health care. **Only you can get you well.** Please remember that. So, if you decide to do three or four of the following therapies – so be it! **You, literally, are the doctor.** What you're reading here is nothing more nor less than "What I would do if I were you."

So, onward........

Exercise With Oxygen Therapy (EWOT)

A message from another prominent member of my great network of cancer researchers and crusaders, **Art Brown**, introduced me to a new therapy. Here's Art's message.

*"The [EWOT] acronym stands for **Exercise With Oxygen Therapy**. A person simply spends about **15 minutes a day** on a treadmill while **breathing pure oxygen**. The oxygen under pressure is what does the trick, being forced into the body while the exercise circulates it around. There is a certain O2 pressure [6 liters per minute] required, certain vitamins to take 1/2 hour ahead of time etc. People seem to be claiming all kinds of wonderful rejuvenating effects for this treatment, especially*

*among the elderly. **Robert J. Rowen MD** of California is one of its strongest proponents. In his former state of Alaska, he was primarily responsible for getting the USA's first state-wide laws enacted that **protect alternative practitioners from relentless attack** by the conventional medical crowd.*

I can't help but think this type of therapy might be highly beneficial to cancer patients. It is well established that oxygen is one of cancer's worst enemies."

Here's more on it from the web site:

http://www.alkalizeforhealth.net/freshjuices.htm

"EWOT

William Campbell Douglass, M.D. highly recommends EWOT. Exercise With Oxygen Therapy (EWOT) is doing light exercise, such as on a treadmill or stationary bicycle, while breathing pure oxygen. EWOT produces the benefits of hydrogen peroxide therapy and you can do it at home. Set the O2 flow at 6 liters per minute, hook the little tube to your nose, and exercise at a moderate pace for 15 minutes while breathing pure oxygen. As part of your cancer prevention and health maintenance program, do this at least once a month. If you are ill with any disease, do EWOT more frequently. In particular, do EWOT after operations, chemotherapy, radiation treatment, x-rays, and burns. Every spa, clinic and health club in the country should offer EWOT."

.....And here's another web site with lots of information on this topic:

http://www.geocities.com/SoHo/Gallery/6412/EWOT.htm

Don't miss Art Brown's own web site. He is a **cancer crusader** who has written a book on the subject and has a very informative web site. Just go to:

http://www.alternative-cancer.net

Essiac Tea

If you have been surfing the Internet at all looking for cancer treatments, you have no doubt heard of Essiac Tea. There are many testimonials of its effectiveness against **all types of cancer**. Here is some background on it.

Essiac tea is a blend of herbs. The formula had been passed up through the Ojibwa medicine men. In **1922**, it landed in the hands of an Ontario, Canada nurse named Rene Caisse. Although Rene was not ill at the time, she asked for the formula in case she might ever need it. Unfortunately and ironically, a member of her family had been diagnosed with cancer and was given six months to live. Sensing that she had "nothing to lose" Rene decided to test the product she came to call "Essiac" (Caisse spelled backwards) tea on her dying aunt. The result was that the woman **went on to live another 21 years**. She eventually died of natural causes.

Inspired by her aunt's success with Essiac tea, Rene Caisse began to offer the remedy's recipe to anyone who asked for it. Eventually, Dr. Charles Brusch **(personal physician to former President John F. Kennedy)** learned of the success of Essiac tea and became a **research partner** with Rene.

The original formula of Essiac tea apparently had eight herbs. The common blend today contains Burdock Root, Sheep Sorrel, Turkish Rhubarb Root, Red Clover, Watercress, Blessed Thistle, Kelp and Slippery Elm bark. Although no formal, clinical studies have been performed to support the merits of Essiac tea, many, many people have **praised its effectiveness** for relief from ailments that include cancer, arthritis, circulatory problems, urinary tract infections, prostate irregularities and asthma.

From **1922 to 1978** Nurse Caisse helped thousands of people with her original herbal formula at her clinic in Bracebridge, Ontario, Canada. Although she **refused payments** for her services she accepted donations to help support her clinic. Rene Caisse dedicated her life to helping others alleviate their pain and suffering with the use of her Essiac® formula.

If you do a search on Google, you will find **34,200** or more references to "Essiac tea." For many years, I did not recommend Essiac Tea as a primary "self-treatment." I have now been introduced to and interviewed a true expert on this subject.

Dale Joy is the **best informed herb expert** I have ever met. She has traveled worldwide researching herbs. She has studied with Native American healers and discovered the "secrets" behind their healing herbs. These "secrets" have to do with the particular **characteristics of the soil** in which the herbs are grown. In short, Dale is the best source for this type of tea I know of. She has helped hundreds of cancer patients recover for over 30 years. Get acquainted with her and what she calls "Modified Native American Tea." You'll find it at her web site:

http://www.herb-t.com

Pau D'Arco Tea

Lots of people have been cured of all kinds of cancer by drinking Pau d'Arco tea (also known as Taheebo tea). Obviously, it is something you should know about.

Roger DeLong is a retired airline pilot who cured himself of cancer using Pau d'Arco tea. He was so convinced it would help people that he set up a simple, inexpensive way for cancer patients to get it. For several years, Roger imported it by the ton and sold it (he even gave it away to those who couldn't afford it). He doesn't do that any more, but he does have a web site with lots of information and a couple of sources he trusts. The cost is about $25 a pound, which is just about a one-month supply. Roger's web site is:

http://www.Pau-d-Arco.com

This tea appeals to me as an inexpensive and effective way to deal with cancer. There are no cautions about interferences with other treatments that I know of. My only caution is to buy it from a **reputable source** like those Roger DeLong recommends so you can be sure of getting the truly effective product.

Protocel/Cancell/Entelev & Graviola

In this section, I'll introduce you to two wonderful cancer survivors. They are both a part of my cancer "network."

Elonna McKibben, Glioblastoma Multiforme Cancer Survivor

There are few cancer survivor stories as dramatic as that of Elonna McKibben. In 1989, Elonna gave birth to quintuplets. Four of the babies survived. When I interviewed Elonna on my web talk radio show, she told me that she had been home schooling her four children and they were just about to complete their senior year of high school.

When her babies were two and a half weeks old, Elonna was diagnosed with a very rare form of nervous system cancer called

Glioblastoma Multiforme, Stage IV. (According to conventional medicine, malignant glioblastomas are virtually always fatal). The diagnosis was the result of a CT scan Elonna was given because of severe pain she had been havng during and after the pregnancy. The scan showed that the source of her pain was a **tumor on her spinal cord** in the thoracic area.

After surgery to remove the tumor, Elonna was paralyzed from the waist down. She was told that the tumor was malignant. The doctors said it was **impossible to remove it** all and that she would not live to see her four babies' first birthday.

She was offered a very aggressive bone marrow chemotherapy treatment or 30 treatments of radiation at very high calibration. The doctors said that this "treatment" would **cause her body great damage** and that her best hope with the treatment was to live another three to six months.

Fortunately for Elonna, her experience with the birth of the quintuplets and subsequent cancer diagnosis had resulted in a lot of media coverage. Elonna and her husband, Rob, received a lot of mail with suggestions for "alternative" treatments. One of those was **Cancell.** Very skeptical at first, Elonna told *Rob "If there was a cure for cancer, don't you think they would be using it instead of letting thousands of people die?"*

Encouraged by Rob, Elonna began taking Cancell on November 12, 1989. She decided to **refuse the conventional treatments** since they offered so little hope. At the end of Elonna's second week on the Cancell, she was admitted back into the hospital because of blood clots and a hemoglobin problem. Fortunately, during her eight days in the hospital, her family was able to bring the Cancell to the hospital and give it to her around the clock.

After several weeks, Elonna began to notice an improvement in her condition. In fact, **18 hours** after taking the first dose of the Cancell, **the "die-off" of the cancer cells began.** She describes the "lysing" (elimination of the dead cancer cells) as follows:

"It literally poured out of me: I threw it up; my bowel movements were extremely loose and stringy and frequent. I lost it in my urine; my nose ran so much I had to keep a tissue with me at all times. I sweated it out profusely; and I had hot and cold flashes and night sweats. When the nurses would give me a sponge bath after a night sweat, the water would be a golden brown color with what they referred to as 'tapioca balls' floating in it."

The lysing symptoms Elonna suffered through were worth it. To everyone's amazement, she had a complete scan of her brain and spinal cord in February, 1990 (only **three and a half months** after she started on the Cancell) and there was no sign of the cancer.

Elonna had to endure a long and painful bout of physical therapy to recover her ability to walk. Today, however, she is **healthy and only uses a walker occasionally.** Elonna has conselled hundreds of other cancer patients by phone at no charge. You can reach her at her home in Ohio. To find her phone number, just go to her web site: http://www.ElonnaMcKibben.com

For the complete story of Cancell (now called **Protocel**), just go to Tanya Pierce's web site: http://www.OutsmartYourCancer.com There, she has two options. You can buy her great book *"Outsmart Your Cancer"* or you can buy the four chapter extract which contains the **full Cancell/Protocel story** – complete with how to take it, what to eat with it, what not to eat with it and many case histories. This extract is an e-book which you can **download for just $9.95.**

Another great book just published by a breast cancer survivor who used Protocel is *"The Breast Stays Put"* by Pam Hoeppner. You can find this one at her web site, which is: http://www.TheBreastStaysPut.com or on Amazon.com. Pam's wit makes this an easy read.

To purchase Protocel (the current name except in Australia, where it is called "Entelev"), just go to: http://www.ProtocelGlobal.com They make no claims about healing cancer. That, of course, is necessary to keep the web site up and avoid harassment by the FDA.

Steve Finney – Protocel & Graviola

Next I would like you to meet Steve Finney. Steve is a Major Account Manager for Cisco Systems. Here is his letter to me:

*"Bill - Just a note of thanks for your 'labor of love' and for your ongoing work despite losing Marjorie. You must be a great friend to many people. I stumbled on your site after searching info on **Graviola**, as the many folks I am involved with who use Protocel (aka Cancell) have recently been made aware of this amazing extract from the Brazilian rainforests."*

[I'll give you some details on Graviola and Paw Paw in the next section.]

Steve's letter continued:

*"I am 39 and was diagnosed with Stage 3 Anaplastic Astrocytoma **brain cancer** about 16 months ago, and after **taking Protocel for only 5 months**, the tumor is absolutely dead and does not enhance whatsoever. Two neuro-oncologists have told me they have never seen my kind of result, and I hear that so often now from others I just take it for granted. I am so*

grateful for Protocel, but I am real excited about it being used **in conjunction with Graviola**. I have heard of 2-3 cases already in which the two were used in conjunction and there was tumor disappearance in **literally days -- serious tumors**.

It would be good to hear from you, but I wanted you to know that I admire your tenacity and love of people to go to the effort to do what you are doing.

 God bless,

Steve Finney,"

Another Protocel Recovery

Here's another letter I received in July 2003 from a reader in Brazil:

"Dear Bill,

Thank you for answering me so fast despite that you are on the road somewhere.

Today I had another meeting with the 'cancer specialist' in Sao Paolo. He said he wants to cut away my lymph nodes on the left side of my neck and then apply radio therapy to burn the tumor. My reply was: No Way!!

I've been on PROTOCEL since June 4 (2003), and the tumor is definitely getting smaller and all my pain that I had for a while is gone. Can you imagine that? In twelve days!

Tomorrow I will be checking in to a natural clinic here where someone will supervise my progress more closely. I will keep you posted on my progress. Thanks again, Bill! You are a real blessing!

Ove"

At last report, Ove is cancer-free and doing fine.

Graviola

My good friend George Freaner, another 88 year old and 25+ year cancer survivor, was kind enough to send me an article on Graviola. You may have heard of this substance before, but I would like to remind you of it, because it is readily available without a prescription and it is quite **inexpensive (cheap!).**

Here's the article. It's from *"The Doctor's Complete Guide to Conquering Cancer,"* published by Agora Health Books of Baltimore, MD:

"Natural Cancer Fighter From the Amazon May be 10,000 Times Stronger Than Chemotherapy

Native medicine men in the Amazon have known about the Graviola tree for centuries. But cancer patients are just starting to learn about the benefits of the natural medicine it provides us with, which some say is more powerful than chemotherapy.

In as many as 20 laboratory studies over the last 30 years, Graviola has been found to selectively kill malignant cancer cells--cells from breast, colon, prostate, pancreatic and lung cancers specifically. In a 2000 study at the Catholic University in South Korea, two chemicals extracted from Graviola seeds showed cytotoxic results comparable to those of Adriamycin, a common chemotherapy drug. Another study, published in the Journal of Natural Products in 1996, found that Graviola killed colon cancer cells at '10,000 times the potency of Adriamycin.' Research at Purdue University found that leaves from the Graviola tree killed six different kinds of cancer cells, showing particular effectiveness against prostate cancer, pancreatic cancer, and lung cancer cells.

Proponents of Graviola report that it is able to selectively kill cancer cells without damaging healthy cells--and without serious side effects. Some users have reported gastrointestinal upset at high doses; this may be avoided, however, by taking Graviola with food. As a nutritional supplement, it is not subject to FDA approval and is available by mail order from Raintree Nutrition; tel. (800) 780-5902. Raintree supplies Graviola leaves, which can be made into a tea, as well as Graviola capsules. The recommended dosage varies from 1 gram to 5 grams of Graviola per day, or six to eight capsules daily. The cost for Graviola is about 20 cents per capsule."

Original Research

I usually don't quote from original research papers. Here's a sample from one on Graviola **which will show you why**:

"They are potent inhibitors of NADH: ubiquinone oxidoreductase, which is in an essential enzyme in complex I leading to oxidative phosphorylation in mitochondria. A recent report showed that they act directly at the ubiquinone-catalytic site(s) within complex I and in microbial glucose dehydrogenase. They also inhibit the ubiquinone-linked NADH oxidase that is peculiar to the plasma membranes of cancerous cells."

And Now – In English

However, here is a quote from that same report on Purdue University's research on Graviola, which is a little more decipherable to us normal humans, and which is **quite significant**.

"In 1997, Purdue University published information with promising

news that several of the Annonaceous acetogenins 'not only are effective in killing tumors that have proven resistant to anti-cancer agents, but also seem to have a special affinity for such resistant cells.' In several interviews after this information was publicized, Purdue pharmacologist Dr. Jerry McLaughlin, , the lead researcher in most of Purdue's studies on the Annona chemicals [Graviola], says cancer cells that survive chemotherapy may develop resistance to the agent originally used against them as well as to other, even unrelated, drugs. 'The term multi-drug resistance (MDR) has been applied to this phenomenon,' McLaughlin says. He explains that such resistance develops in a small percentage of cancer cells when they develop a 'P-glycoprotein mediated pump' capable of pushing anti-cancer agents out of the cell before they can kill it. Normal cells seldom develop such a pump.

'If having this pump was such a good deal, all cells would have it. But all cells don't,' McLaughlin says in a statement from Purdue. 'In a given population of cancer cells in a person, maybe only 2% of the cancer cells possess this pump. But it's those 2% of cancer cells that eventually grow and expand to create drug-resistant tumors.' McLaughlin and his colleagues say some studies have tried to bypass these pumps by keeping them busy with massive doses of other drugs, like the blood pressure agent verapamil. In this way, it was hoped that some of the anti-cancer drugs would enter the cell and destroy it. But this only caused potentially fatal side effects such as loss of blood pressure.

In the June [1997] issue of Cancer Letters, the Purdue researchers reported that the Annonaceous acetogenin, bullatacin, [Graviola] preferentially killed multi-drug resistant cancer cells because it blocked production of adenosine triphosphate, ATP -- the chief energy-carrying compound in the body. 'A multi-drug resistant cell requires a tremendous amount of energy to run the pump and extrude things out of the cell,' McLaughlin says. 'By inhibiting ATP production, we're essentially pulling the plug on its energy source.' But what about the effect on ATP in normal cells? 'Normal cells and standard cancer cells may be able to minimize the effect of this compound because they don't require vast amounts of energy needed by the pump-running cells,' the Purdue researcher says.

'The resistant cell is using its extra energy for this pump as well as to grow, so it is really taxed for energy. When we mess with the energy supply, it kills the cell.'"

A good web site for more info on Graviola is:

http://www.graviola.org

Paw Paw

In the Summer of 2003, I had a conversation with Dr. Jerry McLaughlin. He is the same person I quoted above about Graviola. Dr. McLaughlin had left his research post at Purdue University to join a company called Nature's Sunshine. He explained to me why he did that.

At Purdue, Dr. McLaughlin had worked for **20 years** studying the effect of extracts like graviola, guanabana, soursop and **thousands of others** on cancer cells. He said he had studied 3,500 substances. His research was funded with a $5 million grant from the National Cancer Institute. Despite this funding, the **NCI has never published the results** of Dr. McLaughlin's successful study that you will read below. Are you surprised?

The Paw Paw tree is common in the Midwest U.S. In fact, there is a town in Michigan called Paw Paw. Dr. McLaughlin had spent years studying the various parts of this tree and had found that the twigs, not the fruit, produced the most powerful acetogenins. These are compounds that **regulate the production of ATP**, the energy source in every cell in the human body. For years, Dr. McLaughlin had been searching for one of these acetogenins that would also **inhibit the growth** of "multi-drug resistant" (MDR) cancer cells.

As described in Dr. McLaughlin's study above, most tumors contain a small percentage, approximately 2%, of MDR cells. Chemo is not effective against these cells. After the first round of chemo, if the chemo is effective, all of the cells that are not MDR are destroyed. Since this accounts for the vast majority of the tumor mass, the tumor will **appear to be effectively destroyed**. However, the MDR cells remain and start to multiply. Eventually, a new tumor is formed that is **entirely MDR**. The next time chemo is used, none of the cells will be destroyed because they are **all** MDR. Paw Paw is **even better than Graviola** against MDR cells.

By reducing the ATP, Paw Paw was also able to **reduce the growth of blood vessels** that nourish the cancer cells, a process called "anti-angiogenesis." It also, like Protocel, **reduced the side effects of chemo**. In short, after his many years of searching, Dr. McLaughlin was convinced he had discovered what he was looking for.

To ensure that the manufacture was correct, Dr. McLaughlin went to work for Nature's Sunshine, the company that makes the Paw Paw twigs into a tablet. Even though it is sold by multi-level marketing, Paw Paw is **surprisingly inexpensive**. The price is approximately $30 per month.

Dosage

Take 1 capsule with food four times a day at even intervals. In 2005, Nature's Sunshine had Paw Paw lab tested against all antioxidants – Vitamins C, E, A and beta carotene; Alpha Lipoic

Acid, etc. They found no interference from any of these substances with the action of Paw Paw.

This product is **not a preventative.** While it is effective against viral diseases such as shingles and cold sores, it should not be taken unless there is a specific cellular problem, including, of course, cancer.

Effectiveness

Dr. McLaughlin's studies and others show Paw Paw is effective **only 50% of the time**. Protocel studies show virtually the same 50% effectiveness.

Once again, I need to emphasize that **no one product is a "magic bullet"** that everyone can take and be sure his or her cancer will go away and stay away.

I give you lots of options in this book. Is Paw Paw a good option? I feel it is, particularly for those of you who have had **several forms of chemotherapy** and thus, have probably developed the **multi-drug resistant (MDR) cells.**

VIBE Machine

I was introduced to the VIBE Machine in July, 2005 by Buddy Stairs, one of my readers in Montana. Buddy had owned a VIBE Machine at that time for about 18 months. The stories he told me about his experience healing people with it really got my attention. He was talking about **cancer**, diabetes, arthritis, fibromyalgia and other degenerative conditions. All of them seemed to be responding positively to sitting in front of this machine.

What on earth is the VIBE Machine? Well, I got curious, too. The letters stand for **"Vibrational Integration Bio-Photonic Energizer."** A real mouthful. It had been around since early 2003. While I had heard about it from a couple of readers by e-mail before, Buddy gave me the first real information on results with it.

My wife, Terry and I became curious. We called the home office of the VIBE Machine, which is in Greeley, Colorado and asked for the closest one to us. It was in Tennessee. The owner was a retired Doctor of Osteopathy named Thomas Noll. We loaded a couple of friends in the car and went to see him. We spent the whole day exchanging "war stories" with Dr. Noll and his lovely wife, Katie.

Dr. Noll and Katie, a couple of years before, in 2003, had been to Greeley, Colorado and talked to the inventor. Sceptical when they went, **they came away convinced** and bought one of the machines. They had lots of healing experiences with it that they shared with us.

Terry and I got ours in September, 2005. It was the **first in North or South Carolina.** We had lots of traffic, almost all generated by "word of mouth." Here are a couple of testimonials we've received from our VIBE Machine "customers."

"April 19, 2006

I went to Bill and Terry and the VIBE Machine with the hope of feeling less depressed and more energetic. I have a history of liver challenges and my energy is up and down (mostly down).

I had a mild detox after my first session and after that my energy levels began to rise. I now have a feeling of CORE HEALTH that

I have not had since my teens. Aches and joint pains I have noticed for years are GONE!

In addition, the VIBE Machine has revitalized my cat Boogiebear. He almost died this past Christmas and was dehydrated and listless. He had a blockage. After 3 visits to the VIBE Machine he began acting like a young animal (he is 16 years old) jumping and playing and just being frisky! Now his fur has that healthy luster and he is eating and acting like a young animal. I feel the VIBE Machine saved his life.

Mitch Langen"

"March 28, 2006

I just had to tell you what happened yesterday after I got back home! First, I wasn't fatigued by the drive [she came from 72 miles away] *– actually that may be the understatement of the year! I usually get tired around 3 PM in the afternoon. Not yesterday! I had energy to spare that kept me up until my midnight bedtime! And even then, my thoughts were racing – all positive!*

I injured my thigh muscles back in the summer of '93 when I helped someone lift some long boards that were way too heavy for me. When it happened, I felt something just 'snap' inside my leg. All those 13 years since, I have not been able to sit cross-legged on the floor comfortably – my right leg would stay upright at a 90 degree angle and not bend toward the floor. And even when I would lie down I could not stretch out comfortably. THIRTEEN YEARS! And every single night I had to put a pillow under my right knee so I could lie flat in bed – otherwise, I had pain at the top of my thigh plus sciatic pain across my right buttock.

Well…this morning when I finally got into bed I was laying there for a few minutes before I began to notice that my leg was perfectly straight with no pillow under it and it felt fine. I couldn't believe it! I jumped up out of bed and tried sitting cross-legged on the floor – so far, my right leg now bends at about a 45 degree angle, no problem. Maybe with a few stretches every day, I could actually get it even lower to the floor. I don't want to push it too fast. Right now, even this much seems like a miracle!

I also felt at the top of my thigh, where the muscles always seemed to feel somewhat 'bunched' or tight and rigid – now they are perfectly smooth and there's no pain there anymore whatsoever.

Now do you understand why I have to get back up there today instead of waiting for tomorrow?! <big grin>

See you soon – and thank you so very much for makng the VIBE available! I may have to check into getting one for myself…

Love and blessings,

Cheryl Franks"

Bill Brown's Story

I can't leave the account of the VIBE Machine without sharing Bill Brown's story with you. Here it is, as told by his wife, Willie:

"In September, 2003, Bill was diagnosed with prostate, bone and lung cancer with masses on his adrenal glands. He is a diabetic and has high blood pressure. At the time of the diagnosis, he was gravely ill and unable to undergo chemo or radiation. The doctors gave him 4-6 months to live and told us to go home and get our affairs in order. Bill also had a catheter that was inserted at that time and in a wheelchair.

It was in November that we heard about the VIBE Machine. We looked it up on the Internet. It made so much sense to me and was logical that I told Bill we were going to go the next day, November 21, 2003. We went to Greeley and used the VIBE Machine for the first time [they live in Loveland, Colorado – about 20 miles from Greeley]. *Bill was asked to commit himself on a daily basis for the next 6 weeks. We continued going....*

Bill's tests prior to using the machine got progressively worse and his condition deteriorated...The first test after the use of the machine did not get better, but it did not get worse either. The next test taken showed a marked improvement. Three weeks after he started using the machine he drove the car for the first time in months.

In March, 2004, his doctor sent us a letter telling us his PSA had dropped to 11.1 from over 100 on his previous test....normal being 1-4. During all this time Bill had an indwelling catheter that was surgically removed in June, 2004. Also being on oxygen, his oxygen concentration had gone from 57 to 94 (91 being normal). His blood pressure medication and diabetes medication have been cut in half. In September, 2004, the doctor called and told Bill his cancer was totally inactive. Bill currently is working outside daily and doing a lot of traveling and fishing.

We got our own VIBE Machine on February 9, 2004. We opened our home to those who needed the machine but were unable to pay the fee for its use. We started offering the machine on a donation basis and the response has been increbible. The results with a wide variety of symptoms have been amazing. We have met some of the nicest people and shared their triumphs.

After having been a nurse all my life...seeing and using this alternative method for letting the body heal itself has been an enlightening and wonderful way to end my career in the nursing field.

159

In December, 2004 Bill's doctor notified him that his cancer was totally inactive. He also notified him that he was the first patient in the history of the V.A. Hospital [in Cheyenne, Wyoming] *that had recovered from Stage IV cancer. We feel we owe all of this to the VIBE Machine.*

By Willie (Mrs. Bill) Brown
(Nurse for 50 years – now retired)
Bill Brown (70 years old)
Loveland, Colorado"

Terry and I visited Willie in Loveland in April, 2006. Her daughter now runs their VIBE Machine operation. It is located in a small strip shopping center near their home. We were there on a Sunday for about 3 hours. During that time, all six seats around the VIBE Machine were full every minute with a steady stream of people. Willie says they have **over 100 people every day** using the VIBE Machine.

Incidentally, I couldn't help asking Willie what other changes her husband, Bill, had made in his "lifestyle" during his recovery. She said *"None. He is too stubborn. He won't change anything or take anything. All he will do is sit in front of the VIBE Machine for 8 minutes every day."*

Obviously, I don't recommend you follow Bill Brown's path. If you use the VIBE Machine, it should just be **another tool in your arsenal** of recovery tools. It is a powerful one. However, in our experience, to heal serious conditions like cancer **takes time and patience**. All the VIBE Machine practitioners I've talked to say the same thing. *"Those who come on a schedule get better."* What's a "schedule?" Four times a week or more. If this is too inconvenient, I suggest you use my basic regimen or some other means than the VIBE Machine for your recovery program.

The VIBE Machine is currently being reviewed by the FDA and is temporarily not available. For information on a similar machine, please go to:

http://www.TheQuantumPulse.com

Four More Easy Self-Treatments

I will close this chapter with four more inexpensive and readily available cancer treatments. In Chapter 7, I'll cover those that I DON'T recommend you try, at least not on your own (without a medical professional's supervision).

Red Raspberry Capsules

Why? What are the benefits? Raspberries, like many other fruits, contain **ellagitannins,** compounds that have been shown to have many health benefits, but **raspberries have the most.** These benefits include:

> ➤ Prevention of certain types of cell damage by carcinogens that result in cancer.
> ➤ Slowing of tumor growth.
> ➤ Inducement of natural cell death for cancer cells.

Would you believe that the American Cancer Society has even published information on red raspberries? Knowing what I do about their propaganda, that doesn't give me the greatest feeling of confidence.

Call or e-mail Bob & Jackie Hall for more information on how and where to buy the red raspberry capsules. You can reach them at: Phone: (707) 435-8434 or (800) 964-8276; Email: ellagicacid@gmail.com. Approximate cost: $29.95 for a month's supply of 120 tablets of 1,000 mgs each. They have a special of 6 bottles for $21.95 per bottle.

Artemesinin

In late 2001, two bioengineering researchers at the University of Washington published their discovery of a **promising potential treatment** for cancer. Originating in the ancient arts of Chinese folk medicine, the **wormwood** herb derivative has been used for 30 years to treat malaria.

In the journal Life Sciences, Professor Harry Lai and his assistant Narendra Singh described how they targeted breast cancer cells with artemesinin. The results were indeed surprising. While only 25% of the cells were killed in the first eight hours, **virtually all of them were killed in 16 hours**.

"Not only does it appear to be effective, but it's very selective," Lai said. *"It's **highly toxic to the cancer cells**, but has a marginal impact on normal breast cells."*

Artemisinin works against malaria by reacting with the high concentrations of iron found in the malaria parasite. When artemisinin comes in contact with iron, a chemical reaction ensues, spawning charged atoms that chemists call "free radicals." The free radicals attack the cell membranes, breaking them apart and killing the single-cell malaria parasite.

About seven years ago, Lai began to hypothesize that the process might work with cancer, too.

"Cancer cells need a lot of iron to replicate DNA when they divide," Lai explained. *"As a result, cancer cells have much higher iron concentrations than normal cells. When we began to understand how artemisinin worked, I started wondering if we*

could use that knowledge to target cancer cells."

Lai's work has been funded by a grant from the Breast Cancer Fund of San Francisco. However, artemisinin's **value is hardly limited to breast cancer**. In fact, an earlier study involving **leukemia** cells yielded even more impressive results. Those cells were **eliminated within eight hours**. A possible explanation might be the level of iron in the leukemia cells.

"They have one of the highest iron concentrations among cancer cells," Lai explained. *"Leukemia cells can have more then 1,000 times the concentration of iron that normal cells have."*

Here are web sites with articles that will get you completely up to speed on this interesting substance:

http://www.newswise.com/articles/2001/11/CANCER.UWA.html

http://news.bbc.co.uk/1/hi/health/1678469.stm

http://www.annieappleseedproject.org/artemisinin.html

http://members.tripod.com/~altmedangel/cancherb.htm

Unlike some Chinese herbs, this one has **30 years** of Western scientific studies behind it and is used widely to treat malaria and hemorrhoids (it is anti-inflammatory) and is certainly non-toxic.

Fortunately for you, the University of Washington has patented Dr. Lai's idea. This just means that a pharmaceutical company probably can't pick it up, develop a synthetic form and sell it for **twenty times as much**.

OK, so you're convinced that this substance is an interesting development in cancer treatment. Next question. How do you get it? Good question. I've looked at several sources, including Dr. Donsbach's "Canburst" and Hepalin 25. I have actually ordered one bottle of the **Hepalin 25** (at $56 a bottle for 30 100mg capsules -- a one-month supply) and finished taking it.

Thanks to Dr. Russell K. Griffith, one of my alert readers, here's a very **inexpensive source** for artemisinin.

Artemesinin (100mg, 90 pills) can be obtained from Vitanet (Item no. 72160) for $25.39. That's where I'd get mine now. This is an Allergy Research Group product. Order at:

http://www.myvitanet.com/index.html

Just type "artemisinin" (without the quotes) in their search window. Instead of almost **$2 a day** from the Hepalin 25 source, it works out to **twenty eight cents a day** from Vitanet at the recommended dosage of 1 pill per day.

Thank you, Dr. Griffith!

Beta Sitosterol

If you are a human bean of the male persuasion, I have a suggestion for you. Pay attention to your prostate! Next to heart problems and lung cancer, prostate cancer is the leading cause of death among men. Most of us my age (76) are coping with an enlarged prostate, formally known as Benign Prostate Hyperplasia (BPH).

Thanks to my friend Cy Bursuk, a nutritional consultant in Tucson, I have discovered Roger Mason and his book *"The Natural Prostate Cure."* Every man should read this book. It is the **most complete explanation** of the effect of hormones and supplements on male health in general and prostate health

164

in particular I have ever read. In just 72 pages, he explains **why** your prostate grows larger as you age. He also destroys many of the myths about hormone therapy (for both men and women) and the effects of various substances (including hormones) on your prostate.

What is most interesting about this book is that the author, uniquely among living or dead "experts," has **read EVERY study** on the subject ever published, regardless of language. He did this by reviewing every entry in Chemical Abstracts (known as the "chemist's bible"). This tome contains every published medical article of importance from every scientific journal in the world. In a year of **tough, grinding research**, mostly at the National Institutes of Health Medical Library (the largest such library in the world) in Bethesda, Maryland, he read every one, even getting those **translated** from a foreign language, where necessary. Well-documented conclusions? You bet!

How much does this book cost? $6.95 from amazon.com. The key ingredient Roger Mason recommends for controlling BPH symptoms is "Beta Sitosterol." This substance is needed for prostate health, whether or not you have prostate cancer. One product is ProstatePure Plus from Wellness Partners, Inc. Each of the veggie capsules contains 300 mg of the Beta Sitosterol. A 60-capsule bottle is only $21.99. To learn more about it and order some, you can go to:

http://www.wellnesspartners.com

or call 1-888-779-7177.

A cheaper source for Beta Sitosterol (**150mg**, 40% potency), is Our Health Co-op. It comes in a bottle of 60 for $9.46 (normal retail: $29.95). I trust this source completely. The "40% potency," by the way, does not mean that this product is only 40% as

165

effective as other Beta Sitosterol products. Quite the contrary. At their website, Our Health Coop says "*Our concentrated potency compares to formulations with up to 600 mg of unconcentrated beta sitosterol.*"

Just go to:

http://www.ourhealthcoop.com/

The Final Answer For Me

I took the Beta Sitosterol for about three months. I then tried artemisinin for a couple of months. Finally, in January, 2003, my new doctor (see Chapter 1 above) recommended I try **Prostate Essentials Plus** from

http://www.swansonvitamins.com

I trust Swanson Vitamins as a source. I tried the Prostate Essentials Plus and have **been on it ever since** (over 5 years at this writing). Within two weeks, all my prostate (BPH) symptoms went away – and stayed away. No more getting up several times a night. Once, most nights – occasionally none. No more aching in my lower back. No more urgency or incontinence with my bladder. Nada.

In addition (as if that were not enough), the one time I had an attack of prostatitis (after a very stressful trip back from Europe), I just tripled the dose for two days and the prostatitis went away. A 90-day supply (180 capsules) costs $16.99 from Swanson Vitamins.

[All the prices quoted here are current as of September, 2008. All are subject to change. I just want to give you an idea of the relative prices of these competing products. Check them out for yourself before you buy.]

A Word About PSA Tests

Dr. Thomas Stanley, professor of urology at Stanford University School of Medicine, recently announced at a medical conference:

"We need to recognize that PSA is no longer a marker for prostate cancer. We originally thought we were doing the right thing, but we're now figuring out how we went wrong."

I'd say **it's about time**, Dr. Stanley. It's been reported for years in sources I trust (Dr. Robert Rowen's "Second Opinion" newsletter, for example) that 70% of men with elevated PSAs turn out not to have cancer (a false positive). I'm one of them.

But as bad as it is to get told you may have cancer – or have to undergo a very uncomfortable and dangerous biopsy of your prostate – this is not what got Dr. Stanley to change his mind about the test. What he was concerned about was the alarming number of **false negatives.**

Dr. Rowen says: *"In one recent study, researchers followed 9,459 men who had annual PSA tests. Of this group, 2,950 had test results showing very healthy prostates. But when these 'healthy' men underwent biopsies, a whopping 15% tested positive for cancer! Many had high-grade cancer. And the PSA test missed it in all of them!*

And the incidence of false negatives may be even higher. You see, prostate biopsies are taken by random needle jabs into the gland. [I know. I've had four of them – all negative -- before I got smart!] *No matter how many sticks are made, there's no way to know if cancer lurks outside the needle track.*

Bottom line: Don't rely on PSA to tell you whether or not you have cancer. Focus instead on other diagnostic tests."

If you're still taking one of these PSA tests every 6 months or a year, you might want to consider stopping that. I have. My doctor and I agree that we will run cancer tests (Navarro HCG Urine Test, for example – see above) when I have some symptoms. In the meantime, he (the doctor) does a digital rectal exam (DRE) every six months or so. That's all.

Keep in mind that most men die "with" prostate cancer but not "from" it. Be cautious about both testing (particularly biopsies) and surgery. There are usually better and less invasive ways to treat prostate problems. See my recommended regimen above as one example. It works.

Feel Better Fast!

Let me close out this section on self-treatment with a treatment I have **tried myself**. It works to make you feel better, **no matter what your reason** for feeling bad.

I received this from Phil Dyer, a friend who publishes a newsletter. Phil says it came from the *"Doctor Yourself Newsletter"* by Andrew Saul, PhD. He modeled it from Abram Hoffer, M.D., *"The King of Niacin."*

"If you do not feel well, and I would go so far to say for almost any reason, try this deceptively simple game plan. Go out of your way to promptly get to saturation of the following four key nutrients: niacin, vitamin C, water, and carotene. It is uncomplicated, fast-acting, and very effective on a wide variety

of illnesses."

Certainly, cancer is one of those illnesses. Here's the info Phil is referring to from Dr. Hoffer by way of Dr. Saul:

"1) GET TO NIACIN SATURATION, which is indicated by a mild, warm, pink-eared vasodilation known as a 'flush.' If you are feeling stressed, anxious, depressed, worried or just plain ticked off, try this:

Immediately take 100 to 200 milligrams of niacin (not niacinamide) every ten minutes until you feel warm and happy. If you think this will not work, it's because you have not tried it. While we're at it, Some FEARLESS FLUSH FACTS:

If I had a dime for every person worried about the 'flushing' they experienced when taking large doses of niacin, I'd be a rich man. Niacin flushes are harmless. Some people (including me) enjoy them, especially this time of year, as they are accompanied with some welcome warmth. Dr. Hoffer says that the more niacin you take now, the less you will flush later.

Time needed to see improvement: less than an hour.

2) GET TO VITAMIN C SATURATION, which is indicated by bowel tolerance. That means, take a few thousand milligrams of vitamin C every ten minutes until you get, or feel like you are about to get, diarrhea. This will both clean you out and jump-start your immune system. Vitamin C in quantity is the best broad spectrum antitoxin, antibiotic and antiviral there is.

Time needed to see improvement: less than a day.

3) GET TO WATER AND CAROTENE SATURATION. This can be simultaneously achieved by twice daily juicing a big stack of vegetables, such as carrots and any green or orange vegetable.

Yes, green as well as orange veggies are absolutely loaded with carotene. Yes, you really do have to drink it. What are you afraid of? When's the last time a person died of vegetable overdose? Saturation of carotene is reached when your skin turns a partial-pumpkin, lovely orange-tan color. Called 'hypercarotenosis,' it is harmless. Looks cool, too, much like a suntan. Abundant water intake is guaranteed by abundant juicing. When your tummy is full of juice and you have to urinate a lot, you are at water saturation.

Inside your skin, you are an aquatic animal. Water is good. Veggie juice is better. If you are worried about getting enough trace minerals, relax. Most are amply found in the vegetables.

Time needed to see improvement: less than a week.

If you think I have lost what's left of my marbles, think again. I have never been more serious. When I work with very sick people, the first 'homework' I give is to go flush, reach bowel tolerance, hydrate, and turn orange. Sounds preposterous, doesn't it. But people who do so feel better immediately. Their tests improve immediately. And they learn something of lasting practical value."

Go thou and turn orange!

$$$$ For Your Treatments

Virtually everything we have discussed in this chapter – supplements, most of the tests, etc. – is **not reimbursed by insurance**. Here's some information that may help.

Have you heard of something called **"viatical settlements?"** Neither had I. A viatical settlement is the **sale of a life insurance policy** issued on the life of a person who, in this context, is called a "viator." It is based on a law passed by Congress that went into effect on January 1st, 1997. It is called "The Health Insurance Portability and Accountability Act of 1996.

The person on whose life the policy is written does not have to be the "owner" of the policy. For example, a spouse may be the "owner" of the policy and/or the beneficiary.

What is important is that there are options available to **get money NOW** out of a life insurance policy. That money may be more useful now than after the death of the person on whom the policy is written. What is really ironic is that the money obtained in this manner **may actually extend the life** of the "viator" for many years. [Hint: Don't let the people buying your policy know how effective the "alternative" treatments are that you will be taking!]

The procedure, which amounts to selling the policy to a third party, covers all types of life insurance policies -- term, whole life, "key-man" policies, buy/sell agreement policies and so on. Basically, someone is **buying the life insurance** benefit at something less than the full amount payable on the covered person's death (50-85%, depending on life expectancy).

For "seniors" 70 or older, the policy can be sold **regardless of the insured's health**. Generally, the proceeds of the sale are **tax-free**. Obviously, some paper work and time is involved, so **don't delay**. If you are interested in further information, here's a toll-free number to call to get a brochure from one company that specializes in this (it's not the only one). The number to call is (888) 321-9057. It's a company called Viatical Settlement Professionals, Inc. in Richmond, Virginia. They also have a web site (who doesn't?). It's at: http://www.vspi.com

CHAPTER 6
CLINICS

In this chapter, I will give you some information on clinics in the U.S., Mexico and Europe which I've become familiar with. Generally, if you can afford it, I recommend you seek out one of these clinics. The concentrated attention they give you during your stay at the clinic can be life saving. The comprehensive "take-home" advice you leave with is also priceless. The best, including those I mention here, dedicate themselves to follow-up with you until you are cancer-free, and even after that.

Immune Recovery Clinic

In late March 2004, my wife and I visited the Immune Recovery Clinic in Atlanta, Georgia. My portion of this trip was paid for by one of my readers in Venezuela, Andres Kese. Andres was very impressed with the healing treatment for his advanced prostate cancer he received from this clinic. He was so impressed that he offered to pay my way for a visit there so I could help publicize them.

We were impressed. The staff is enormously well qualified and their work with cancer patients is quite successful. While we were there, we met one of my readers, who had responded to an earlier article on this clinic I had written and gone there for treatment. She had arrived with Stage IV breast cancer and was making great progress. She had been there 10 days and was ecstatic with the quality of the treatment and the attitude of the staff. She is now cancer-free.

Dr. Richard Kinsolving, (another Ph.D.) has a world-wide reputation as an expert on the immune system. He meets with the patients daily during their 3-week stay to educate them about healing and staying healed. Ed Bradford is the CEO and Clinic Director. They have various other experts on the staff, including one in Chinese Medicine.

Their motto, which I completely believe, is *"Cancer and chronic disease cannot exist in the presence of an intact immune system."*

The treatment here usually consists of a three-week stay. Patients sleep at a very comfortable (and reasonable) motel three blocks away. Follow-up varies, but usually involves a visit or two several months apart after the initial treatment.

The cost? $4,500 flat fee per week, payable at the beginning of each week at the clinic. They price it this way for two reasons. First, they don't want their choice of treatment for each patient (which is unique) to be influenced by cost; and second, if they find that they cannot treat you, the expense can be limited. The good news is that they work very hard with your insurance company to get you reimbursed for most of this cost. Ed Bradford, who does most of this work for the patients, says he recovers 60% of the cost, on the average.

To explore this clinic further, I suggest you either call Ed Bradford at (800) 336-3533 or (770) 455-6100 or visit their web site at:

http://www.ImmuneRecovery.net

New Hope Medical Center

One of my readers, Ethan Bauch, was treated for a lymphoma in his neck at New Hope Medical Center in Scottsdale, Arizona in late 2003. He had become disgusted with the ham-handed nature of the treatment he was getting from his conventional doctors.

Ethan was delighted with the treatment at New Hope. He spent three weeks there, which is typical. He is cancer-free now.

New Hope uses a variety of regimens for their patients. For the past two years, for example, they have been using **stem cell therapy**. Dr. Fredda Branyon, who I interviewed recently on my web talk radio show, says they limit the patients to 6 to 10 at one time. This insures that each one gets very individualized attention. The charge is $3,900 per week. Some insurance companies will reimburse part of this, some as much as 80%.

Contact Dr. Fredda Branyon. Their contact address and phone number is:

New Hope Medical Center
8945 E. Calle Buena Vista
Scottsdale, AZ 85255
(480) 473-9808

Duke Integrative Medicine

On March 30th, 2007, I heard a very interesting presentation from Dr. Tracy Gaudet at a conference in Greenville, South Carolina on "Integrative Medicine." She is an M.D. (OB/Gyn) but a very unusual one. After studying "alternative" medicine under Dr. Andrew Weil and others and studying Chinese herbal treatment, she has been put in charge of Duke University's Integrative

Medicine Center on the Duke campus in Durham, North Carolina.

Dr. Gaudet showed the attendees some pictures of a beautiful and well-designed 27,000 square foot facility made possible by a $12 million donation from a wealthy Reiki Master. She described a variety of services which are unique, in my experience. For example, here's how she described one of their service options:

"We act as your personal physician advocate, overseeing all of your health needs and coordinating care and communciation among specialists and providers. Often, we coordinate and collaborate in your health from a distance, assuring that all of your health needs are being addressed, and drawing from the best of conventional and alternative practices. Our clients experience therapies such as acupuncture and hypnosis, and learn self-care strategies like stress reduction, nutrition, healthy cooking, and meditation and put them into practice by living them with us. When our clients return home, we encourage them to work with our health coaches to bring these new strategies and skills to bear in their daily lives."

You can contact Duke Integrative Medicine at (866) 313-0959 or check out their web site at:

http://www.dukeintegrativemedicine.org

Mexican Cancer Clinics

Several years ago, when I first began researching cancer causes and cures, I heard about all the clinics in Mexico. Frankly, I felt less than enthused about them. Probably quacks and charlatans preying on cancer victims, I thought.

Wrong!!

After reading dozens of testimonials written by ecstatically grateful cancer patients cured in Mexican clinics, I have become a believer. Read some of the stories of dedicated physicians like Drs. Clark and Gerson, who have been hounded out of this country by our FDA/AMA "gestapo," and opened clinics in Mexico. You will become a believer, too.

Here is some information from an article by Art Brown titled "Mexican Hospitals - Some of the World's Best for Alternative Cancer Care." It was written in January, 2001. The entire article can be found at The Cancer Cure Foundation's web site: http://www.cancure.org

"Most people do not tend to think of Mexico as a haven for cancer treatment, but there are approximately 40 clinics and hospitals there offering some of the finest alternative medical treatments for cancer today. They vary in size from one-doctor operations to modern, multi-story, full-service hospitals with an extensive range of doctors on staff. Most are located close to the Mexican/American border across from San Diego, California. Some are even within walking distance of the border that avoids the need to wait in line in your car for half an hour at the border to clear customs. Although a passport or visa is not necessary, valid identification identifying your country of birth, such as driver's license, is required. [This has changed recently. **Take your passport!**]

Why do patients go to these clinics and hospitals?

In Mexico, the political system is such that the government credits and inspects clinics and hospitals, but does not attempt to get in between the doctor and patient. In short, it leaves doctoring to doctors. This means they are free to use treatments from countries around the world which have proven successful in battling cancer. They can also develop and perfect their own treatments and immediately use therapeutic breakthroughs as soon as they become available.

Not so in the United States where cancer treatments are usually limited to varieties of chemotherapy, radiation and surgery. This is unfortunate as there are about 100 other useful, non-toxic cancer treatments, almost all of which have well-documented scientific evidence to support them.

Having freedom-of-choice regarding treatments, Mexican doctors have been able to develop their skills in using both conventional and alternative therapies, schooling their staffs in them and setting up appropriate patient care facilities. In addition, over the years they've learned which treatments, or combination of treatments, work best for which conditions.

An unusual 'sub-specialty' in cancer care has arisen in Mexico out of all this. Although hospitals there get patients from around the world, the majority comes from the United States (This is another reason they locate close to the border.) These people typically have received conventional cancer treatments where they live without success. Frequently they are very sick with bodies severely weakened by surgery, radiation or chemotherapy. As a result, Mexican clinics and hospitals have become accustomed to helping patients with extra burdens. Not only must they treat end-stage cancer for people coming to them as a last resort, which is a task far more difficult than in the earlier stages, but they must also undo the damage done by conventional 'therapies.'

Best of the Best

Not all clinics and doctors in Mexico are worthwhile of course. We recommend only the best of the best. That is, those we feel are the most experienced, reputable and reliable - large or small. We have toured many facilities, talked to the staff, are familiar with their operations and talked to patients. Typically, they've been around for many years. One in particular has treated over 100,000 cancer patients with alternative treatments in the last 35 years. A record like that speaks for itself. (Call us to arrange a free consultation with a doctor from that particular hospital.) For more information and recommendations, phone (800) 282-2873, or (805) 498-0185 M-F, 9-5, Pacific time."

You may want to look into tours of these clinics. There are at least two agencies in California who offer organized tours. Detailed information on each of these is in the book "Third Opinion." Here is some brief contact information:

Private Cancer Clinic Tours
P. O. Box 530218
San Diego, California 92153
Phone: (619) 475-3834
Contact person: Roberto Rodriguez

Tour of Tijuana, Mexico Clinics
P. O. Box 4651
Modesto, California 95352-4651
Phone: (209) 529-4697
Contact person: Frank or Rosario Cousineau

Frank Cousineau has published an e-book called "Cancer Defeated." It is a complete description of the best Mexican cancer clinics. Here's how he describes the information in his book:

"So I've prepared a special step-by-step guide called 'Cancer Defeated! How rich and poor alike get well in foreign clinics' It has names, addresses, phone numbers, websites and detailed descriptions of selected clinics…."

You can order this book by clicking on this link:

http://www.cancerdefeated.com

Other Clinics in the United States

Frank Cousineau (see above) has also published a great e-book (with Andrew Scholberg) on outstanding alternative cancer clinics in the U.S. Frank is available as a "coach" to help you find the right one for you. The e-book is called "Cancer Breakthrough USA!" and is available at:

http://www.CancerBreaktrhoughUSA.com

In the back of this e-book is contact information to get Frank's "coaching," if you feel you need it. Obviously, the first step is to get the e-book and read it. I was impressed with the various choices of clinics in the USA which Frank and Andy have given you. These clinics practice **true alternative medicine** (unlike Cancer Treatment Centers of America, etc.).

German Cancer Clinics

Andrew Scholberg, the same gentleman who helped Frank Cousineau write the above two e-books, visited six German cancer clinics in the Spring of 2008. His e-book on these clinics is outstanding. It seems every one of these clinics use a very effective technique used **nowhere else in the world**. It is a form of hyperthermia using (short wave) radio frequencies which penetrate well into the body.

Andrew mentions many celebrities who have used these clinics to recover. The doctors he interviewed at these clinics certainly sound like they have a truly holistic approach to healing.

If I had cancer, I'd certainly study this e-book and investigate several of these German clinics. To get the e-book, just go to:

179

http://www.GermanCancerBreakthrough.com

Las Mariposas Clinic of Spain

The only clinic in Europe on which I have positive "first person" information from an actual cancer survivor is Las Mariposas Clinic in Spain. It is located in Torremolinos, near Malaga on the Costa del Sol. This clinic is the only one in the world I have heard of which offers you a money-back guarantee if their treatment does not work.

Contact information and a huge amount of information about their treatment are available at their web site in Spanish and English. You will find it at:

http://www.MariposasClinic.com

Here is an e-mail I received from Tom Brubaker, a reader in Palma de Mallorca, Spain:

"Hi Bill,

Thank you very much for your last newsletter, which I have printed out for my neighbor, and which I am going to use for its information and links. I went to see Dr. Raymond Hilu at the Mariposas Clinic in Torremolinos and spent a week there in a very nice four star hotel for 65 Euros a day because it is off season.

Raymond is a dedicated person and I am sure he treated me both generously and carefully, having done two blood tests, before and after treatment. In my case, he used a mechanism that combines the Rife therapy with three other applications, based on laser directed to the acupuncture points. He gave me Cell Food from Nu Science in Lancaster, California and B complex, B12, Linseed oil, (He had spent some time with Dr. Johanna Budwig,) and other supplements. I have also taken three separate weekly treatments twice a day of Rife and Hulda Clark applied by a friend of mine who is a healing practitioner according to German law and living here."

At last report, Tom is cancer-free and doing fine.

CHAPTER 7
OTHER TREATMENTS YOU
SHOULD KNOW ABOUT

"First, do no harm"
Hippocrates (400 B.C.)

There are a whole slew of cancer treatments out there touted by **credible experts** and **not-so-credible amateurs**. Many of these are quite effective **IF** a medical professional at a clinic where you are under constant supervision administers them. Others are just not proven to be effective or they are inferior to other readily available treatments or they are too expensive.

You will probably hear about each of these at some time during your journey. It is just as helpful, in my opinion, for you to know about those that are not as effective or which require professional supervision as those above in the self-treatment chapter. The goal is to make you an **expert "co-doctor."**

Laetrile/Amygdalin/Vitamin B17

A good example is Laetrile. I believe that Laetrile has helped thousands of cancer patients since it was first discovered in 1953. First, some background.

World Without Cancer

The best book I have found on the subject of Laetrile is *"World Without Cancer"* by G. Edward Griffin, first published in 1974. It has been through **many updates** including 15 printings since then -- the most recent in **March 2000**. He has exhaustively researched the **history and science of Laetrile (B17).** He has personally researched the reason the FDA banned Laetrile. Once you read this book, you will no longer believe in the **"protection"** being provided you and me by agencies like the FDA, the American Medical Association (AMA), and the American Cancer Society (ACS).

If you go to the Cancer Cure Foundation web site, which is:

http://www.cancure.org

click on "Cancer" and type in B17 at the "Search By Word" page, a number of articles will come up. The first one covers both sources of the B17 (Laetrile) capsules and apricot seeds and clinics all over the world that use this as part of their cancer cure protocol, complete with phone numbers.

Edward Griffin documents the suppression of Laetrile and its advocates for what it is -- a **conspiracy** to prolong the superb profits of the **"cancer industry."** The book contains very persuasive evidence that **Laetrile works**. This includes many case studies with the **names and hometowns** of the individuals. I will quote just one to give you an idea of the power of this book:

"WILLIAM SYKES

In the fall of 1975, William Sykes of Tampa, Florida, developed lymphocytic leukemia plus cancer of the spleen and liver. After removal of the spleen, his doctors told him that he had, at best, a few more months to live.

Although chemotherapy was recommended -- not as a cure but merely to try to delay death a few more weeks -- Mr. Sykes chose Laetrile instead. In his own words, this is what happened:

'When we saw the doctor a few weeks later, he explained how and why Laetrile was helping many cancer patients, and suggested that I have intravenous shots of 30 cc's of Laetrile daily for the next three weeks. He also gave me enzymes and a diet to follow with food supplements.

In a few days I was feeling better, but on our third visit the doctor said that he could no longer treat me. He had been told that his license would be revoked if he continued to use Laetrile. He showed my wife how to administer the Laetrile, sold us what he had, and gave us an address where more could be obtained.

The next week I continued on the program and was feeling better each day. One afternoon the doctor from Ann Arbor called to ask why I had not returned for the chemotherapy. He said I was playing 'Russian Roulette' with my life. He finally persuaded me to return for chemotherapy, so I went to Ann Arbor and started the treatments. Each day I felt worse. My eyes burned, my stomach felt like it was on fire. In just a few days I was so weak I could hardly get out of bed... The 'cure' was killing me faster than the disease! I couldn't take it any longer, so I stopped the chemotherapy, returned to my supply of Laetrile and food supplements, and quickly started feeling better. It took longer this time as I was fighting the effects of the chemotherapy as well as the cancer...

In a short time I could again do all my push-ups and exercise without tiring. Now, at 75 years of age [20 years after they said I had only a few more months to live], I still play racquet ball twice a week."

In a letter to Edward Griffin, the author of "World Without Cancer," dated June 19, 1996, Mrs. Hazel Sykes provides this additional insight:

"After Bill had conquered cancer, a doctor came to him one day. (This was an M.D. who gave chemotherapy in a well-known hospital.) He wanted to know how Bill had conquered his cancer because his wife was quite ill with cancer. Bill said: 'Why don't you give her chemotherapy?' His answer was: 'I would never give chemotherapy to any of my friends or family!' He was not the only doctor who came to Bill with the same question."

The Doctor is "In"

Many M.D.s have weighed in with opinions on the use of Laetrile to control cancer. Here are a few examples:

In 1994, **P. E. Binzel, M.D.** published his results from treating cancer patients with Laetrile between 1974 and 1991. He used a combination of intravenous and oral Laetrile. Intravenous doses started with 3 grams and worked up to 9 grams. After a period of months, oral Laetrile, 1 gram at bedtime, was begun in place of the injections. Dr. Binzel also used various nutrient supplements and pancreatic enzymes, as well as a low animal protein, no junk food diet as part of his regimen for cancer patients.

Out of a series of 180 patients with primary cancer (non-metastasized or confined to a single organ or tissue), 138 were still alive in 1991 when he compiled his treatment results. At that time, 58 of the patients had been followed for 2 to 4 years, while **80 had a medical follow-up from 5 to 18 years**. Of the 42 patients who had died by 1991, 23 died from their cancers, 12 from unrelated causes, and 7 died of "cause unknown."

Among his **metastatic** cancer patients, 32 of 108 died from their disease, while 6 died of unrelated causes, and 9 died of "cause unknown." Of his 61 patients still alive in 1991, 30 had a follow-up between 2 and 4 years, while **31 had been followed for 5 to 18 years.**

Binzel's results are impressive. Some of the individual patients discussed in his book were still alive (and well!) **15-18 years** after their initial Laetrile treatment. Binzel also notes that **none** of the cancer **diagnoses** were made by him, a small town, "family doctor". All patients had diagnoses from **other physicians**. Many had already suffered the **ravages of standard "cut-burn-poison"** (surgery/radiation/chemotherapy) medicine before being given up as **hopeless** cases by orthodox doctors.

His book is called *"Alive and Well,"* by P. E. Binzel, M.D. published by American Media in 1994 at Westlake Village, California.

Manuel Navarro, M.D., former professor of medicine and surgery at the University of Santo Tomas in Manila wrote in 1971: *"I…have specialized in oncology for the past eighteen years. For the same number of years I have been using Laetrile-amygdalin in the treatment of my cancer patients. During this eighteen year period I have treated a total of over five hundred patients with Laetrile-amygdalin by various routes of administration, including the oral and the I.V. The majority of my patients receiving Laetrile-amygdalin have been in a terminal state when treatment with this material commenced.*

It is my carefully considered clinical judgment, as a practicing oncologist and researcher in this field, that I have obtained most significant and encouraging results with the use of Laetrile-amygdalin in the treatment of terminal cancer patients, and that these results are comparable or superior to the results I have obtained with the use of the more toxic standard cytotoxic agents."

[This is the same Dr. Navarro who founded the Navarro Clinic which still performs the HCG Urine Cancer Test (Chapter 5 above). The clinic is now run by his son, Efren Navarro, M.D.]

This quote is from the book *"World Without Cancer"* by G. Edward Griffin, mentioned above and in Appendix A to this book.

*"**Dr. Ernesto Contreras** of Tijuana, Mexico has used Laetrile as a cornerstone of his cancer practice since 1963. He remarks that 'For the prevention of cancer and the maintenance of remission, there is nothing as effective as Laetrile…Its non-toxicity permits its use indefinitely while surgery, radiation and chemotherapy can only be administered for a limited time…the majority of cancers that occur more frequently, such as cancers of the lung, breast, colon, ovaries, stomach, esophagus, prostate, and the lymphomas, are much helped by Laetrile.'"*

This next quote is from a book called *"An Alternative Medicine Definitive Guide to Cancer,"* published in 1997 by Future Medicine, Tiburon, California.

Dr. Hans Nieper is a world famous oncologist in Germany. He is the developer of the standard anti-cancer cytotoxic drug cyclophosphamide. In 1970, he co-authored a brief paper on Laetrile with Dean Burk, in which he stated that *"…in the treatment of cancer, the active principle of nitrilosides is to be used mainly in prophylaxis* [prevention] *and early protective therapy… On the other hand, the complete atoxicity* [lack of toxicity] *of this method of treatment, which is maybe nothing else but a rediscovered natural principle, permits the unlimited use of this substance."*

This quote is from a paper entitled *"Problems of Early Cancer Diagnosis and Therapy,"* published in 1970 in the German periodical Aggressologie, Volume 11, page 1-7.

In 1972, Dr. Nieper told reporters while in the U.S.: *"After more than 20 years of such specialized work, I have found the non-toxic Nitrilosides – that is, Laetrile – far superior to any other known cancer treatment or preventive. In my opinion it is the only existing possibility for the ultimate control of cancer."*

This last quote is from *"World Without Cancer,"* mentioned above.

Many of the physicians whose anti-cancer programs are detailed in **"The Alternative Medicine Definitive Guide to Cancer,"** mentioned above, also report positive Laetrile results as part of their cancer treatment programs. **Robert Atkins, M.D.**, the "Diet Revolution" guru, noted that *"Amygdalin appears to neutralize the oxidative cancer-promoting compounds such as free radicals… It's just one more key component keeping cancer from growing or spreading. Contrary to what people have said about Laetrile…it should be considered an effective, entirely safe treatment for all types of cancer."*

Why Not Self-Treat With Laetrile?

In the face of the above evidence and doctor's ecommendations, why don't I include Laetrile/Amygdalin/Vitamin B17 in the "Self-Treatment" chapter of this book? Here are the reasons:

Laetrile's use to cure cancer needs to be part of a complete protocol of diet, enzymes, exercise and supplements, AND supervised by a medical professional.

For example, a proper level of zinc in the body is required for Laetrile to be effective. It doesn't work without adequate Vitamin C. Vitamin A interferes with its effects. A build-up of vitamins, enzymes and a proper diet for at least two weeks before starting the Laetrile treatment is necessary. A full stomach lessens the effect of Laetrile. Finally, the dosage of Laetrile requires injections along with capsules. The reaction must be monitored closely and the dosage adjusted over a period of at least three weeks after the body has been prepared properly to receive the

Laetrile. Definitely not a "do-it-yourself" operation.

Other treatments, which I do suggest to you as universally necessary for cancer patients include things you can do yourself with no supervision. These include: immune system boosters, flaxseed oil/cottage cheese, Vitamin C with L-Lysine and L-Proline, barley pills, Paw Paw, EWOT, red raspberry capsules, artemisinin, enzymes, Ph testing, a radically different diet and a vitamin/mineral supplement. (See Chapter 5 above.) None of these interfere with any other treatments you may be taking.

In Summary

Laetrile (amygdalin) is an effective preventative and treatment for cancer. It should be used under the supervision of a qualified medical professional.

Shark Cartilage

Another treatment you should be familiar with, but which I would wait to discuss with your chosen CAM medical professional is shark cartilage. Beginning in October 1991, Dr. Williams has published **numerous articles** on this subject in his *Alternatives* newsletter.

I feel the best way to familiarize you with this option, however, is to quote from an article by the **discoverer** of shark cartilage, **I. William Lane, Ph. D.** When I called Lane Labs, the sole source for both MGN-3 and shark cartilage, to check on their relationship to Dr. Lane, I got his son on the phone. He said that while his father had no financial interest in Lane Labs, he did consult with them frequently on the products they produce, including shark cartilage.

As you may remember from Chapter 5 above, the FDA managed to shut down Lane Labs briefly in 2004. They are back in business now. Their web site is:

http://www.lanelabs.com/

I will give you information here on their shark cartilage because I think it is an interesting case study of the harrowing nature of the fight to bring natural treatments to us.

Dr. Lane began studying shark cartilage as a potential cancer therapy in September 1983. **Using his own funds**, he conducted studies in Belgium and Mexico. Studies in the United States were too expensive. However, in September 1992, he aroused the interest of the **Cuban Health Ministry**. They invited him to do a study on **non-responsive terminal** cancer patients. Here is an excerpt from an article he wrote in 1995 for *Alternative & Complementary Therapies -- A Bimonthly Publication for Health Care Practitioners:*

*"The Cubans agreed to provide me with 29 patients and a team of five oncologists, seven nurses, and the best possible follow-up. The Cuban study has, as a result of **extensive coverage** and story by **Mike Wallace and '60 Minutes,'** become a legend.*

*These 29 patients were all **unable to get out of bed**, and all were designated as **terminal and dying**. They had **failed to respond** to all available conventional cancer therapy. I almost gave up on the first day. I felt that my **chances** with such advanced patients were **nil**, a belief shared by the Cuban oncologists, headed by Lt. Col. Jose Menendez, M.D.*

*There were 10 different tumors represented including five in the **prostate**, six in the **breast**, five in the **central nervous system**, two in the **stomach**, two in the **liver**, two in the **ovary**, two in the* *uterus, two in the **esophagus**, two in the **tonsils**, and one in the **urinary bladder**. By the **fifth week** I learned via my telephone and fax that the Cuban team was becoming **very hopeful**. I was due to visit on the sixth week.*

*Earlier, I had been contacted by **CBS and '60 Minutes.'** The station wanted to go ahead with the story, which the station had **initially looked upon as a scam**. For the visit on the sixth week of therapy, I, thus, was accompanied by **David Williams, D.C.**, the editor of the health newsletter **Alternatives**, five people from '60 Minutes' (including the **producer Gail Eisen**, who was **medically oriented** and initially **very negative** about the story), and Charles Simone, M.D., a consultant who I had asked to help me evaluate the results. It was clear to all of us that a number of the patients were **already responding**.*

*Except for Dr. Simone, who joined us at 16 weeks, this same group visited again at **11 weeks** and again at **16 weeks**. We were joined at this time by **Mike Wallace**, who stayed with us in Cuba for three days to review the results and to do filming.*

*At this time, the Cubans had added Fernandez Britto, M.D., a **world-class pathologist**, to the team. He showed, for the first time, **autopsy pathologic slides** that demonstrated the action of the shark cartilage in stimulating the rapid growth of fibrin tissue **replacing and encapsulating the cancer cells**. His slides, which now include **'before' and 'after' biopsy** slides, add materially to the explanation of how and if shark cartilage works.*

*'60 Minutes' later showed **X-ray pictures** along with blood work records to Eli Gladstein, M.D. , of the University of Southwestern Texas for collaboration; Dr. Gladstein **confirmed the findings** and he did so **without knowing that shark cartilage was the therapeutic agent**.*

*The '60 Minutes' team was so **excited** about these results that it broadcast the show **within 10 days** after their tape was finished; and they **showed it twice**, something that is rarely done. The team also promoted the story each time for four days prior to the broadcast.*

*Fortunately, this show had a budget that was large enough to truly **study the effects**, **see the patients**, and then **report on the positive results** they themselves observed. The **National Institutes of Health** (NIH), on the other hand, surprisingly, **never took the time to hear the whole presentation, see the slides, talk to me, or talk to the interested doctors.**"*

*"Of the original **29 terminal patients**, nine **(31 percent) died of cancer**, all within the first 17 weeks; **none have died of cancer since**; **six** others have died of accidents, heart failure, or other **natural causes**; 14 **(48 percent) are completely well and cancer-free after 34 months** (almost three years) as of June 15, 1995. After the 60 gm/day of shark cartilage for 16 weeks, these patients went to the **maintenance dose** of 20 gm/day, which appears to have been **keeping them well** for almost three years. With **stage IV** cancer patients, this is very impressive, even incredible, even if one or two patients might have been at stage III rather than stage IV at the outset.*

*All cancers had been **biopsy-confirmed**. The head Cuban oncologist, Dr. Menendez, told me recently, 'In my history as an oncologist, I have never seen or experienced anything like this response with shark cartilage.' "*

Here are Dr. Lane's own words on his discovery.

"I am proud that I was willing to put my own money on the table to develop the shark cartilage therapy, and I will defend the results as will others who have seen the responses.

Peer review *is a cornerstone of our system but other results, if well documented and supported, should not just be* **discarded and ridiculed**.

The **poor results** *with conventional cancer therapy should suggest that* **any new therapy** *that seems promising should be investigated, especially if it is* **inexpensive, nontoxic, and noninvasive**. *In these times of uncontrolled health costs, and the* **cancer epidemic** *that does not seem to be abating, all possibilities deserve attention."*

Summary

Shark cartilage in both powder and capsule form is available from Lane Labs (see web site above). I don't recommend self-treatment with it. My concern has to do with dosage and monitoring. For both, you need the advice of a medical professional.

Dichloroacetate (DCA)

In February, 2007, I published an article "DCA – The Latest Cancer Cure" in my "Cancer-Free" newsletter. I quoted an article by David McRaney, Executive Editor of "Student Printz" on DCA. Here's an excerpt from that article:

"Scientists may have cured cancer last week.

Yep.

So, why haven't the media picked up on it?

Here's the deal. Researchers at the University of Alberta in Edmonton, Canada found a cheap and easy to produce drug that kills almost all cancers. The drug is dichloroacetate, and since it is already used to treat metabolic disorders, we know it should be no problem to use it for other purposes.

Doesn't this sound like the kind of news you see on the front page of every paper?

The drug also has no patent, which means it could be produced for bargain basement prices in comparison to what drug companies research and develop.

Scientists tested DCA on human cells cultured outside the body where it killed lung, breast and brain cancer cells, but left healthy cells alone. Rats plump with tumors shrank when they were fed water supplemented with DCA.

Again, this seems like it should be at the top of the nightly news, right?

Cancer cells don't use the little power stations found in most human cells - the mitochondria. Instead, they use glycolysis, which is less effective and more wasteful.

Doctors have long believed the reason for this is because the mitochondria were damaged somehow. But, it turns out the mitochondria were just dormant, and DCA starts them back up again.

The side effect of this is it also reactivates a process called apoptosis. You see, mitochondria contain an all-too-important self-destruct button that can't be pressed in cancer cells. Without it, tumors grow larger as cells refuse to be extinguished. Fully functioning mitochondria, thanks to DCA, can once again die.

With glycolysis turned off, the body produces less lactic acid, so the bad tissue around cancer cells doesn't break down and seed new tumors.

Here's the big catch. Pharmaceutical companies probably won't invest in research into DCA because they won't profit from it. It's easy to make, unpatented and could be added to drinking water. Imagine, Gatorade with cancer control.

So, the groundwork will have to be done at universities and independently funded laboratories. But, how are they supposed to drum up support if the media aren't even talking about it?

All I can do is write this and hope Google News picks it up. In the meantime, tell everyone you know and do your own research."

My Comments

I really appreciated about eight of my wonderful loyal readers bringing this new development to my attention back in early 2007. I did some more research on it just before finishing this latest update to my book. The best web site for information on DCA is: http://www.TheDCASite.com.

You'll find lots of information there, including a source for ordering the DCA. Unfortunately, because of a visit by the FDA to Jim Tassano, the man behind the above web site, in July, 2007, they are **not able to ship it to orders from the U.S.** They can ship it to other countries.

You'll find many testimonials from cancer patients at this web site. In the forum where people chat about DCA, I found an interesting comment:

"If you look up Dr. Budwig's diet of flaxseed oil and low fat cottage cheese (1950's) you will see that normalization of the mitochondrial/cell membrane potential is the theory that lies behind it…The similarities between the process attributed to DCA and that to flaxseed oil/low fat cottage cheese in the re-establishing the correct potentials is very interesting."

Is it possible that by eating your FO/CC smoothie every day (see Chapter 5 above), you are **accomplishing the same thing you would by taking DCA**. It certainly seems likely just from the "Phoenix rising from the ashes" effect I've heard about from **hundreds of "late stage" cancer patients** eating their FO/CC.

With the DCA unavailable in the U.S. (thanks to our diligent FDA), if I were you, I'd redouble my efforts to make the FO/CC a part of my daily regimen. Read about DCA, though. It is a classic case of a simple, harmless substance which has great promise for healing cancer being suppressed in the U.S.

Grape Juice

Grape juice is one treatment I was considering putting in the "self-treatment" category. Here is an account from a "true believer."

"My experience with this grapeseed diet is good. About 5 years ago I came across it in a book called 'Magnetic Therapy' by Abbot George Burke, 1988, DeVorss & Company, P.O.Box 550, Marina Del Rey, CA 90294

In it the author describes the Grape Cure as suggested by Fred Wortman, of Albany, Georgia, and told by Joseph F. Goodsavage, and printed in this book, 'Magnetic Therapy.'
.

'The doctors,' Mr. Wortman said, 'refused to operate when they discovered the condition of my bank balance.' Being a wide reader, he remembered a simple remedy for cancer that was given in a book by a 'Mrs. Brandt,' and looked it up. It was rather involved and cumbersome to follow, so he reduced it to its essentials, took the cure and was completely cancer-free within a month.

Wortman then had his experiences published in the 'Independent' and received hundreds of replies. Over two hundred cancer sufferers reported complete cures-total recovery. The grape treatment cured lung cancer in two weeks, he reported. Cancer of the prostate took a little longer--about a month. Only four cases of leukemia (cancer of the blood) were treated, but the judicious usage of grape juice cured them all.

The Self Treatment

Start the treatment like this: Begin with twenty-four ounces of (dark Concord) grape juice the first thing in the morning. Do not eat until noon. Take a couple of swallows every ten or fifteen minutes (don`t gulp it down all at once). After twelve o` clock, live the rest of the day normally, but do not eat anything after 8 o`clock in the evening....Food seems to carry off the curative agent in the grape juice, which may be Magnesium, so stick to the fast between 8 PM and noon the following day.

Keep this up every day for two weeks to a month...The dark Concord grape juice treatment is reported to be nearly 100% effective.'

Later on Wortman collected information on four hundred cases treated successfully this way. (All this is found on pages 52 and 53 in the above named book.)

When I took it myself for general health several times, I felt great, lost some weight (about five to eight pounds over a month) and it was easy to do. I am grateful for having found this 'diet,' because I remember the old Italians always saying, 'Se vuoi stare bene devi fare una mangiata di uve per due settimane, ogni tanto.' {If you want to stay (be) healthy you have to eat a lot of grapes, [only grapes], for a two week period every now and then.} Hmmm....they seemed to know a lot back then, eh?...

197

*The danger of this diet may be that the Concord grape juice (or any dark grape juice) may be contaminated with pesticides, hormones (GMO), and/or may be grown in soil where there is fluoride in the water that is absorbed by the grapes. To minimize this risk, either buy organic grape juice, Kosher grape juice, or know the farm where the grapes are grown and make your own grape juice. (Also, **excess sugar** is now found in a lot of grape juices made from concentrates, 'to make it taste good'/supermarket brands... etc.)*

This search for good grape juices could be a bit awkward at times but can be more effective as a self-help treatment and certainly worth the extra effort. Good luck."

Caution

The above seems to indicate that this common staple might be worth a try. It's food, after all. The caution I advise is the result of the following e-mail I received a few weeks after first publishing the above in one of my newsletters.

"Hello,
My name is Bob Rabel. My wife has been battling ovarian cancer for three years now. We've tried many supplements and diet changes, some successful, some not. I appreciate your newsletters greatly. However, you might want to tell your readers what my wife experienced. She tried the grape juice therapy in your newsletter. She used pure organic 100% Concord grape juice just as the therapy advised. Many know that cancer cells grow 3 to 5 times faster in high levels of glucose. We were a little bit skeptical about the fructose content in grape juice. Turns out we were correct. Her tumor marker almost jumped 100%. In her 3 1/2 years it has never jumped higher than 25%. Keep in mind this was just one month's time. A word of caution might be given with this therapy because, in my opinion, the grape juice was the culprit.

Sincerely,

Bob Rabel"

Thank you, Bob. I can only hope the effect on your wife's condition was temporary. Because of the **adverse effect of sugar on cancer**, I'd suggest if you want to try the grape seed treatment, you order "Grape Seed Extract," 50mg, 60 capsules for $7.47 from www.ourhealthcoop.com

Cancer Is A Fungus – Dr. Tullio Simoncini

Many of you have heard by now of the Italian oncologist, Dr. Tullio Simoncini and his theory that cancer is just a fungus – namely **candida.** Here is an excerpt from an article in my August 2nd, 2007 "Cancer-Free" newsletter on this subject:

"This may be one of the most important pieces of information about cancer I've shared with you in the last seven years of writing this newsletter.

Got your attention?

OK. Finally, last week, I learned that the work of Dr. Tullio Simoncini, the Italian oncologist, had been translated into English. You may have heard of him. He's been in the news lately. He has been healing cancer patients using sodium bicarbonate (baking soda) for some number of years now. You can learn about his work and buy his book, "Cancer Is A Fungus" in printed form at:

http://www.curenaturalicancro.com

Get this, now. What he's saying is that the microbe that gets into the cell and causes it to become a fermenting (cancer) cell is nothing other than candida. And treating it requires nothing more than getting baking soda next to the area with the cancer cells and the cells die. That may be a bit over-simplified, but not much.

I've ordered his book but haven't received it yet. There are some interesting videos at the web site and a lot of other information. For example, here is the list of cancers which he says he has treated successfully with the sodium bicarbonate:

Oropharynx cancer
Stomach cancer
Liver cancer
Peritoneal carcinosis
Intestinal cancer
Cancer of the spleen
Tumour of the pancreas
Bladder tumour
Prostate tumour
Pleura tumour
Tumours of limbs
Brain cancer
Lung cancer
Breast cancer
Skin cancer

Impressive list, no? His information on procedures is getting out to the true holistic physicians. I only have space to quote two. Here is an excerpt from an e-mail from Dr. Dana Flavin. Dr. Flavin is a cancer doctor from Connecticut:

"Dr. Simoncini is reversing cancers with 5% solution of baking soda in the artery at the tumor. 6 days on, 6 days off. After 4 sessions the tumors are gone. Breast, pancreas, colon, brain, lung, etc. He also treats peritoneal carcinomatosus, with intra-peritoneal therapies. He has the patients rotate ¼ of a turn every 15 minutes for one hour to cover the whole area. He says it is

getting rid of fungi. I think it is also adding back oxygen by pulling off the hydrogen and adding the CO2, as well as creating an environment that is not palatable for fungi. Tumors hate oxygen and so do fungi...they said it worked better with cisplatin and guess what? Cisplatin is toxic to fungi. Isn't this almost the most ironic thing you ever heard of? Sometimes I just smile and think how simple God has made things and how complicated we have interpreted it."

Dr. Flavin recommended another web site:

http://www.cancerfungus.com

There you'll find several videos, including videos of Dr. Simoncini's lectures on the topic and some patient testimonies."

My Comments

Like everyone else, including several other physicians I've heard from, I was impressed with Dr. Simoncini's findings. I have **three reservations** about you seeking out someone to heal you using his baking soda procedure:

First, finding a **physician properly trained** is not easy. As you will see in the videos above, treating internal tumors in the lungs, etc. requires the insertion of a catheter into an artery and guiding it to the site of the tumor with the help of a radiologist. Not simple and **certainly very expensive**.

Second, the treatment concentrates on **killing the cancer cells**. As you may have noticed, my emphasis is on revising your lifestyle to make your body hostile to cancer cells. Any treatment which concentrates on killing the cancer cells tends to **take away the focus from that process**. You heal cancer by drastically and permanently changing your lifestyle, not aiming your artillery at the tumor, which is just a symptom.

Finally, there are **many other theories about fungus and cancer.** For example, Dr. Hamer (German New Medicine) says that fungi are part of he body's natural healing process. They go to work to clean up the cancer cells when signalled to do so by the brain. His theory, which is backed up by thousands of brain CT scans, would explain why all autopsies of cancer patients show fungi in and around the cancer tumor.

Cesium Chloride

An item I read recently reminded me of the difficult time we had trying to get my former wife's doctor to control her pain. I finally discovered a pain clinic at our University of Texas Health Science Center. A wonderful doctor there got it under control using MS-Contin, a form of time-release morphine. That was in 1994.

But now, there may be a much better solution - a natural, non-prescription substance called cesium chloride that controls severe cancer pain.

Here's the excerpt which caught my attention:

Beginning on page 313 of the book *"Painfree in Six Weeks"* by Dr.Sherry Rogers:

"The Pain of Terminal Cancer

No pain is scarier than that of terminal cancer. And you will be as amazed as I was to discover that researchers have shown that it can be terminated in some cases in less than one day, in fact within a matter of hours with a simple over-the-counter mineral.

This is in spite of these cases being resistant to morphine and other standard narcotic treatments. And even more excitingly, persistent use of this common mineral has been part of a program where inoperable or metastatic end-stage tumors have even shrunk and totally disappeared.

Cesium (pronounced seez' e um), is the non-toxic mineral, that in some folks has stopped cancer pain within 12-24 hours in many cases. And when combined with other minerals and vitamins, all non-prescription, it has caused complete disappearance of tumors within 3 months to two years in some cases (again, it depends on each person's total load and individual biochemistry).

Why haven't we heard of it? The same reason the media does not feature the stories of folks with end-stage cancer who have totally healed themselves of all cancer and metastases with diet and other non-prescription treatments. There is no money in it and, more importantly, it does not deify and empower those who want total control over your pain and health.

Normal cells get transformed into cancer cells via the combination of (1) environmental chemicals that generate free radicals and (2) nutrient deficiencies from a poor diet. Even government studies show that 95% of cancer is caused by diet and environment. The free radicals in turn damage genetics and other regulatory mechanisms and membranes. With damaged cell membranes, as one example, oxygen can no longer readily enter the cancer cell, but glucose or sugar can. In fact, sugar is like fertilizer for cancer cells.

To better understand how cesium works, let's look briefly at the inside of a cancer cell and see what else makes it different from normal cells. Normal healthy cells live, breathe and make energy via a process called aerobic (with oxygen) metabolism. They rely on oxygen. The cancer cell does not rely heavily on this process,

203

having switched its chemistry to a fermentative process using much less oxygen, but lots of sugar (anaerobic). Now you can see why taking a box of candy to a cancer patient is like pouring gasoline on a fire. Sugar and alcohol are like fertilizer for cancer."

Cesium chloride (the only form suitable for human consumption) is available from:

http://www.TheWolfeClinic.com/cesium.html

They have tablets in various sizes -- 10 mg, 50 mg, 100 mg, 500 mg and 1,000 mg. A bottle of 100 of the 500 mg tablets, for example, costs $75. A bottle of 100 of the 10 mg tablets costs $29.95. The pain relief from this substance is, quite obviously, not limited to terminal cancer patients.

They cannot ship this product to an address in Canada. They can ship to the U.S. Shipments to other countries will depend on customs regulations.

There is a **minimum order of three bottles** at one time. They can be of various sizes. They ship them in 4-6 business days or overnight, if you ask for it. The clinic is located in British Columbia, so they are in the Western time zone. You can reach them at (800) 592-9653 or (250) 765-1824.

Caution

A reader with some experience with this substance warns that you have to take it **with food**. She said it can cause **stomach bleeding and irritation** otherwise. You should also take it with **potassium** and **other supplements** to avoid heart palpitations.

Another reader (an RN) with some experience with it warned not to **try self-treatment**.

Based on the above, I suggest you try cesium chloride **only** under the supervision of your own medical professional.

PolyMVA

Several readers have alerted me to a substance called PolyMVA. From what I have been able to learn from my own research, I'm convinced this is a valid substance, both as a **preventative and a self-treatment**.

Poly-MVA (MVA = minerals, vitamins and amino acids) is a non-toxic antioxidant composed of alpha lipoic acid and the element palladium. Developed in the U.S. by Dr. M. Garnett, the discoverer of the Second Genetic Code, it has already proven effective against many degenerative diseases, including cancer.

My research on the Internet turned up the Advanced Brain Tumor and Cancer Poly-MVA Hospital in Tijuana, Mexico as one of the first treatment centers for this therapy. Starting 20 years ago with treatment of brain tumors, they have now determined that the therapy is just as effective for **virtually all types of cancer**.

For lots of testimonials and to order it online, check out both of these sites:

http://www.polymva.net

http://www.polymvasurvivors.com

The Catch

One of those survivors is a personal friend now. She arranged for me to talk to her Businesswoman's Luncheon group in Austin, Texas.

So, what's the catch? Why wouldn't this qualify as a good self-treatment? In a word – **expensive!!** An 8 oz. bottle costs **$330.** A month's supply is **four** of these. There are much simpler and cheaper alternatives, which, in my opinion, are equally effective.

OTHER CANCER TREATMENTS

In this section, I will summarize all the other "alternative" cancer treatments I have found in my years of research. In studying these, ask yourself the obvious question: "Why hasn't at least one of these inspired the official cancer research community to explore it further?"

Rife/Bare Electrical Resonance

Cancer therapy and electrical frequency resonance met first in the 1930's. **Dr. Royal Rife** built the device. In 1934, **physicians** from the University of Southern California conducted **clinical trials**. They used it on 16 cancer patients at the Scripps Ranch in California. The results? Within 60 days, 14 of the 16 people were pronounced **cured** of their cancers. The remaining two people were pronounced **cured** within the next 60 days.

The Rife Device, using electrical resonance, had the ability to **destroy or devitalize** specific cells and microorganisms. It is alleged to have the ability to remove **cataracts** from patients' eyes.

James E. Bare, D. C., picked up the torch. He published a **book in 1997**. The book, *Resonant Frequency Therapy -- Building the Rife Beam Ray Device,* includes instructions on **how to build the device**. Dr. Bare claims that anyone can build it in about **four hours**.

Since learning about the VIBE Machine and watching it work, I have had little faith in the more primitive "Rife machines" (self-built or manufactured) which try to duplicate his cancer treatments.

"The Cure For All Cancers" (?)

Hulda Regehr Clark, Ph.D., N.D., is a **remarkable person**. I'm sure you will find her book, *The Cure for All Cancers*, as fascinating as I did. Published in 1993, this book documents not only 100 cancer cases she treated personally but also instructions on building an **electronic device** to replicate her tests.

Dr. Clark's hypothesis is that parasites or intestinal flukes cause all cancers. Her Doctorate is in biophysics and cell physiology. After working on Canadian government research projects for eleven years, she began private consulting in 1979. In 1990, she put together her theory on **cancer cause and cure**.

The parasites Dr. Clark claims to have isolated come from all manner of **toxins** in our food, our water, our cosmetics and even the **fillings in our mouths**. Eating out of Styrofoam containers is a "no-no." In fact, she lists multiple everyday items which contain traces of 33 **"unnatural chemicals"** harmful to our bodies (arsenic, barium, cobalt, lead, radon, tin and so forth).

The **constraints** she suggests on your life to avoid all these **"cancer causers"** are so severe, most of us would simply throw up our hands in despair, as I did. For example, you must stop smoking (good idea!); change your **copper** water pipes to **plastic**; remove all **chemicals** from your house; board your **pets** with a friend; get rid of any possible **asbestos** sources (hair dryer and clothes dryer); have your house tested for **radon**; remove all possible **formaldehyde** ("if your bedroom is paneled, move out of it and keep the door locked."); remove all possible **arsenic** (wallpaper glue, roach killer, lawn chemicals, etc.); check your home for exposed fiberglass; and check your **gas** heat and gas water heater for **leaks**.

She's not done. You also have to remove all **metal fillings** from your mouth and have infected teeth removed and **"cavitations"** on your jaw by an **oral surgeon**. I agree with her that **toxins leeching out of our teeth** are the **unrecognized (by the "establishment") cause** of many diseases. [See Chapter 5 on "Root Canals."]

Dr. Clark's theories about the cause of cancer are not that "radical." She mentions **cell "mutations",** just as Dr. Roizen [in Chapter 2] did. Her contention is that she has discovered the CAUSE of the mutations. It is **"intestinal flukes"** which migrate primarily due to the presence in our bodies of isopropyl alcohol.

Dr. Clark has **added much** to the understanding of **causes and treatments** for cancer. No study of alternative/complementary treatments is complete without looking at her work. Like other pioneers, she has been **persecuted** by our medical "system." In 1999, the FBI **arrested her** in San Diego and extradited her to Indiana where she was tried for "practicing medicine without a license." After she had spent **several months in jail**, all **charges were dismissed** in a trial in April, 2000.

Dr. Clark now operates one of the many cancer clinics in Tijuana, Mexico. You can get the full story on Dr. Clark, including her brief stint in jail in 1999 at:

http://www.drclark.ch/

Included at this web site are **over 100 detailed testimonials** of cancer patients healed using her methods.

In summary, there are cheaper, better (in percentages of healings) and easier methods for getting cancer-free than those Dr. Clark recommends.

"On Our Own Terms" and "Wit" – An "Aside"

In 2000 I saw Bill Moyers' six hour TV special on **death and dying** called *"On Our Own Terms."*

The intimate interviews with dying people and their caregivers and doctors were **extremely moving** for me. It brought back **many memories** of my own experience with my former wife, Marjorie. It also caused me a great deal of **frustration** to see the **needless suffering and death** that is occurring every day because of ignorance of what you are reading here.

Another truly moving time for me in 2006 was watching the **Emma Thompson movie "Wit."** If you have cancer, you need to see this movie.

None of the alternative therapies we are covering here actually **shorten your life**, as do most chemotherapy and radiation treatments. They do not **destroy your immune system**, as do most chemotherapy and radiation treatments. They are **non-invasive and non-toxic**. They don't kill patients, even when they don't heal them.

"Most cancer patients in this country die of chemotherapy," observes Dr. Alan Levin of the University of California Medical School. *"Chemotherapy does not eliminate breast, colon or lung cancers. The fact has been documented for over a decade…Women with breast cancer are likely to die faster with chemotherapy than without it."*

As you read about the various therapies in this book, remember that they are included here because they have healed at least some cancer patients. Unlike conventional medicine, I don't define "healed" as **survival for five years**. I define "healed" as being able to return to a **normal lifestyle and maintain it indefinitely through a normal life expectancy.**

Antineoplaston Therapy

The following is a **classic example** of how our medical system reacts to a discovery that may fundamentally alter current beliefs. This negative reaction parallels the **public punishment** of medical pioneers down through the ages.

"The body itself has a treatment for cancer," says Dr. Stanislaw Burzynski. The Polish-born physician-biochemist, based in Houston, Texas, discovered that a group of **peptides** (short chains of amino acids) and amino-acid derivatives occurring naturally throughout our bodies **inhibit the growth of cancer cells**.

In his view, these substances are part of a biochemical defense system **completely different** from our immune system. Unlike the immune system, which protects us by destroying invading agents or defective cells, the biochemical defense system **reprograms**, or corrects, defective cells. It carries "good" information to abnormal cells, instructing them to develop normally. Does this remind you of the "proofreader" cells we discussed above? Our bodies are **wonderfully complex** creations.

Dr. Burzynski named these peptides **anti-neoplastons** because of their ability to inhibit neoplastic, or cancerous, cell growth. He discovered that cancer patients have a **drastic shortage** of these compounds in their bodies. Blood samples of advanced cancer patients reveal only 2 to 3 percent of the amount typically found in healthy individuals. By simply reintroducing the peptides into the patient's bloodstream, either orally or intravenously, he brings about **tumor shrinkage or complete remission**. In many cases, just weeks after the start of treatment, tumors have shrunk in size or disappeared.

Since the Burzynski Research Institute (BRI) opened in 1977, Dr. Burzynski has treated some 4,000 cancer patients, most of them in advanced stages. There is no doubt from the peer-reviewed literature he has published **(150 scientific papers)** that his treatment works, at least for some patients. In fact, he holds **20 patents** for antineoplaston treatment covering **16 countries**. Dr. Burzynski advises that antineoplaston treatments are neither effective against all types of cancer nor for all patients.

Burzynski's breakthroughs are being eagerly pursued abroad. Clinical studies are underway in **Japan, Poland, Great Britain, Italy and China**. In September, 1990, the Burzynski Research Institute entered into a letter of intent with Ferment, a major Soviet pharmaceutical firm, to conduct **clinical trials** with antineoplastons on cancer patients **in Russia**.

How has his work been received in the United States by the cancer "establishment?" Well, you probably guessed it. His work has been dismissed as **quackery** by such interlocking government agencies as the Food and Drug Administration and the American Cancer Society. Oncologists, when asked by patients about Dr. Burzynski, respond that he **hasn't published anything**.

The FDA **filed suit** against Dr. Burzynski in March 1983 in an attempt to drive him out of business. It ordered Burzynski and his Institute to stop all further research, development, manufacture, and use of antineoplastons. A federal judge allowed the doctor to continue his research and treatment **within Texas** but ruled he could not ship the drugs across state lines.

In July, 1985, **FDA agents** and federal marshals, armed with an illegal search warrant to look for vague "violations," **raided** the Burzynski Research Institute and seized over 200,000 **confidential documents**, including private medical records. They went through Dr. Burzynski's personal correspondence and rifled his briefcase. The federal officers loaded **eleven** of his filing cabinets onto their truck in an outrageous violation of his (and patients') constitutional and civil liberties. Dr. Burzynski sued the FDA for the return of his records, but all the documents remain in the FDA's hands to this day.

The Texas State Board of Medical Examiners tried to revoke Burzynski's medical license in 1988 on hairsplitting technical charges that had **no connection** with the quality of care he provides. Hundreds of letters of support were sent to the board by Burzynski's patients and their families and friends. The following letter from a Midwestern teenager was typical:

"I am 13 years old and I have a 7 year old brother. We love our father very much. Thanks to Dr Burzynski's treatment, my father's tumor has stopped growing. All of the doctors in my home state of Missouri said there was no cure for my father's disease. Dr. Burzynski gave him a chance for life again. Please don't take that away from us."

There's more to this story. If you want the **complete story** and several more case studies, please get the book *"Options – The Alternative Cancer Therapy Book"* by Richard Walters, copyright 1993 published by Avery. It is available from amazon.com.

The bottom line is that to the American medical monopoly, Dr. Burzynski and his therapy are a **threat** in at least three ways. First, if his theory about a biochemical defense system separate from the immune system is correct, the biology textbooks will have to be rewritten. His theory is **revolutionary** in its implications and he has **impeccable credentials**.

Second, although he is an alternative healer, Burzynski **plays by the rules**. He publishes his findings openly and widely in the **peer-reviewed medical literature**. This makes it harder, but obviously not impossible, to smear him as a quack.

Third, and most important, his **safe, non-toxic** cancer treatment, with its tremendous promise, is perceived as a threat by the **mega-billion-dollar cancer business** with its vested interests in toxic chemotherapy, radiation and surgery. Orthodox doctors and the huge drug companies would not welcome a safe, relatively inexpensive cancer cure – such as naturally occurring peptides, an herbal brew, or something similar – that can't be marketed to reap **super profits**.

Contact information for Dr. Burzynski's Houston clinic is in Appendix A to this book.

My Personal Experience

My information about the Burzynski therapy is second hand. A close personal friend who I will call "Paula" (not her real name) had a hysterectomy on September 17th, 2001. The pathology report showed endometrial cancer cells in the lining of the uterus. In a few days after the operation, she began taking magesterol, a hormone.

Recovering nicely, she began taking several CAM products -- MGN-3, beta glucan, shark cartilage and acidophilus. She was feeling good.

Paula and her husband read lots of literature on cancer, including my first book "Cure Your Cancer." They decided to try the Burzynski Clinic in Houston, Texas (in spite of my warning, by the way). After sending Paula's records a couple of weeks before, they visited the clinic at the end of October 2001. Their experience was **anything but positive**.

After waiting one hour beyond their appointment time, they were seen by one of the physicians. Paula commented to him that they probably wouldn't have had to wait an hour if she had been **Jane Seymour or one of the other celebrities** whose pictures filled the walls of the fancy clinic building.

Their interview with the physician proved that he had not looked at Paula's records. This, of course, bothered them.

Paula had a discussion with Dr. Burzynski, himself. She asked him if he had statistics on the treatment's success with ovarian cancers like hers. He said they **didn't have enough** to compute valid success rates. She also asked him for names of CAM-sympathetic doctors in San Antonio. He said he would get her some names.

As for Paula, she was given a large number of pills called PBN (sodium phenylbutyrate). She was told to begin with 1 every two hours, six times a day. That was to be built up to **NINE every two hours**. They said to continue taking the MGN-3, but stop taking the beta glucan and acidophilus because they interfered with this treatment.

By the time she reached the **FIFTY FOUR** pills per day level, Paula was **very sick**. She was so nauseous, she could not hold down either the Burzynski pills or any other medication or food. She called the Burzynski Clinic. The physician said stop taking the PBN until the nausea went away, then begin at a lower level again.

When Paula asked for the names of CAM-competent doctors that Dr. Burzynski had promised her, the physician said Dr. Burzynski was out of town and he didn't know anything about that.

Paula passed away early in 2003. Her husband said she was just unable to control her cravings for unhealthy food.

The **statistics** that Burzynski publishes are **not very impressive**. For example, they showed that as of July 2001, the **"objective response"** rate for both colon and breast cancer was **57.2%**. The rest had either "stable disease" or "progressive disease." Objective response means **"complete response, partial response or substantial decrease in tumor size."**

The cost: **$4,500 PER MONTH**. They handle only outpatients. The payment seems to cover only **office visits** (about every six weeks, in Paula's case) and the **medication**. While a few insurance companies will reimburse for the treatment, Medicare will not.

Obviously, I'm not a great fan of the Burzynski treatment. I would consider it only as a **last resort for brain tumors**.

The 714-X Compound and Gaston Naessens

A French biologist now living in Canada, Gaston Naessens developed a non-toxic treatment for cancer and other degenerative diseases. Called 714-X, the compound is an aqueous solution of nitrogen-enriched with camphor molecules. Camphor is a **natural substance** derived mainly from the camphor tree of East Asia. The camphor-nitrogen compound is injected into the body's lymphatic system. It is said to strengthen the patient's ravaged immune system, which then **rids the body of disease**.

Based on **forty years** of microscopic and biological research, Naessens' treatment has restored health to **hundreds** of cancer patients, many of them **diagnosed** by orthodox doctors **as terminal**. Many patients experience dramatic benefits, including **relief of pain**, improved appetite and weight gain, increased strength, cessation of vomiting, and feelings of well-being. A course of treatment consists of daily injections for at least three 21-day periods, with a 3-day rest between each period. For advanced or metastatic cancer, an average of seven to twelve periods is recommended. Patients can be taught to **self-administer** the treatment.

Again, detailed information on the science of this remedy and case studies are available in Richard Walters' book *Options*, mentioned above. You can also find there detailed information on **sources** for the substance and treatment. I will not elaborate on it further, because I believe other substances mentioned above are much more readily available and at least as effective.

It's no surprise that the Canadian medical establishment hounded Naessens. Quebec's medical-drug complex has dismissed his treatment as worthless. Nevertheless, Canadians can obtain 714-X through the emergency drug branch of the federal government for patients suffering from degenerative diseases (cancer, AIDS, etc.)

His research shares much **common ground** with that of other cancer researchers. His discovery of pleomorphic (form-changing) organisms in the blood **tracks with the immune theories** of Virginia Livingston, M.D. (see below) and the electromagnetic frequency generator developed by Royal Rife (see above).

As I write this, Gaston Naessens is 84 years old. One of the primary goals of the **Independent Cancer Research Foundation (ICRF)** I have founded (with four other cancer researchers) is to document and preserve the 714X compound. If possible, we will make it available through a non-profit outlet like Our Health Co-op. For details on the ICRF and its goals, see below.

Revici Therapy

Dr. Emanuel Revici has developed another original approach to the treatment of cancer. His non-toxic chemotherapy uses **lipids** and other substances to correct an imbalance in the patient's chemistry. Lipids – organic compounds such as fatty acids and sterols – are **important parts of all living cells**.

The Romanian-born physician, who practiced in New York City, had applied his wide-ranging discoveries for over **sixty years** to the treatment of cancer. The great majority of his cancer patients were in **advanced stages** of the illness. Many years after receiving his treatment, some of these patients were in remission with **no signs of active cancer**.

Commenting on Revici's 1961 book, *Research in Physiopathology as a Basis of Guided Chemotherapy with*

Special Applications to Cancer, Dr. Gerhard Schrauzer, a leading authority on selenium, wrote, *"I came to the conclusion that Dr. Revici is an innovative medical genius, outstanding chemist and a highly creative thinker. I also realized that few of his medical colleagues would be able to follow his train of thought and thus would be all too willing to dismiss his work."*

Dr. Revici tailored his treatment to the individual. One patient, a forty-three year old man, was diagnosed with an invasive, high-grade of cancer of the bladder at Memorial Sloan-Kettering Cancer Center in September 1980. They said, *"The only way you can be treated is if we **take your bladder out** and give you a **colostomy** on the side."* He said no. The patient visited Dr. Revici in October and went on his therapy. He has had no other treatment. In 1987, he returned to Sloan-Kettering for a cystoscopy, which revealed him to be **cancer-free**.

Another patient, a twenty-nine year old woman, was operated on at Memorial Sloan-Kettering in October 1983 for a chordoma, a **brain tumor**. The tumor was incompletely removed, and she was given a course of **radiation therapy**. Her condition progressively worsened during the twelve months following the surgery. Dr. Revici first saw her in May 1984. At the time, she was confined to a wheelchair with **limited function**. She started the Revici program. She subsequently had **two babies** and functions well. Her only problem is that she **walks with a cane**.

Revici's non-toxic cancer therapy never received fair testing or funding in the United States. That should come as **no surprise** to any of you who have read this far. His methods have been formally studied and put into practice in **France, Italy and Austria**. He was a distinguished physician who graduated **first in his class** at the University of Bucharest.

The American media portrayed him as a quack that should have been **put out of business**. The American Cancer Society put Revici's therapy on its Unproven Methods blacklist in 1961. In 1984, the State of New York tried to revoke his medical license **permanently** on the grounds of deviation from standard medicine, negligence, incompetence, fraud, the use of unapproved experimental drugs, and similar charges. After **four years** of struggle, Revici won in July 1988. The court decision allowed him to **continue treating cancer patients.**

To save his license, Revici's patients and several medical civil-liberties groups undertook **extensive lobbying** at the state capitol. At the federal level, New York Congressman Guy Molinari held an **all-day hearing** in March 1988 to address the Revici matter and the whole field of alternative cancer therapies. Dr. Seymour Brenner, , a respected radiation oncologist in private practice in New York, testified **on Revici's behalf**.

Dr. Brenner had investigated a number of patients in very **advanced stages** of cancer, **incurable** by orthodox means. Revici had put **each of them** into long remissions. Dr. Brenner had an **independent panel of pathologists** confirm the diagnosis and stage of illness prior to each patient's initial visit to Revici. He testified that his personal findings strongly suggested Revici has a cancer treatment **deserving further study**, and he proposed that the **FDA conduct such an evaluation.**

In a letter to Congressman Molinari, Brenner outlined a protocol in which a **panel of doctors** would monitor cancer patients placed on alternative therapies. All of these patients would have been **declared untreatable** by conventional means. The letter contained **detailed case histories** of ten advanced cancer patients whom Revici had healed.

It is now almost **fifty years** since Revici developed his non-toxic chemotherapy. An open-minded, unbiased evaluation of it by the cancer "establishment" has **never been done**. Once again, the cancer industry succeeded in suppressing an alternative non-toxic treatment that showed promise to **replace, or at least enhance**, toxic chemotherapy and radiation.

If this type of suppression and ridicule of promising cancer cures interests you, you will find twelve painstakingly documented cases in Daniel 's book *"Politics In Healing."* I strongly recommend it to you.

Fighting Cachexia With Hydrazine Sulfate

Cachexia (pronounced ka-KEK-si-a) is the wasting away process that kills **two-thirds** of all cancer patients, including my former wife, Marge. Hydrazine sulfate **dramatically reverses** this process. It is an inexpensive drug, with **no side effects**. It has a clinically documented anti-tumor action. It causes malignant tumors to stop growing, to reduce in size, and, in some cases, to disappear.

About **half** of all patients who take hydrazine sulfate experience **weight gain**, restored appetite, **extended survival time**, and a significant **reduction in pain and suffering**. Many patients report an increase in vigor and strength and the disappearance of symptoms of the disease, along with feelings of well being and optimism.

While hydrazine sulfate may not be a sure-fire cancer cure (and what is?), **large-scale clinical trials** suggest that it affects every type of tumor at every stage. It can be administered **either alone or in combination** with cytotoxic chemotherapy or radiation to make the cancer more vulnerable to the standard forms of treatment.

Dr. Joseph Gold discovered the effects of hydrazine sulfate in **1968**. Cancer has two principal devastating effects on the body. One is the **invasion** of the tumor into the vital organs and the destruction of the organs' functions. To the general public, this sounds like the most common cause of cancer death. In fact, it accounts for **only 23%** of the cancer deaths each year.

The other devastating effect of cancer is **cachexia**, the terrible wasting away of the body. It means weight loss and debilitation. In cancer, as in AIDS, patients **die from the accompanying illnesses**, which they would otherwise survive if not for the wasting syndrome.

"In a sense, nobody dies of cancer," notes Dr. Harold Dvorak, chief of pathology at Beth Israel Hospital in Boston. *"They die of something else – pneumonia, failure of one or another organs. Cachexia **accelerates that process of infection and the building-up of metabolic poisons**. It causes death a lot faster than the tumor would, were it not for the cachexia."*

But what causes cachexia? Cancer cells **gobble up sugar** ten to fifteen times more than normal cells do. The sugar consumed by the cancer cells is generated mainly from the liver, which **converts lactic acid into glucose**. (Normal cells are far more efficient users of glucose, which they derive from the food we eat, **not from lactic acid**.)

When cancer cells use sugar (glucose) as fuel, they **only partially metabolize it**. Lactic acid – the **waste product** of this incomplete combustion – spills into the blood and is taken up by the liver. The liver then **recycles** the lactic acid (and other breakdown products) back into glucose. The sugar is consumed in ever-increasing amounts by **voracious** cancer cells.

The result is a vicious cycle, what Dr. Gold calls a **"sick relationship"** between the liver and the cancer. The patient's **healthy cells starve** while the cancer cells **grow vigorously**. Some healthy cells even dissolve to feed the growing tumor.

To break this sick relationship, Dr. Gold reasoned, all he needed was to find a **safe, non-toxic drug** that inhibits gluconeogenesis (a big word meaning the liver's recycling of lactic acid back into glucose). In 1968, he outlined his theory in an article **published in Oncology**. *"The silence was deafening,"* he recalls.

A year later, by remarkable coincidence, Gold heard biochemist Paul Ray deliver a paper explaining that **hydrazine sulfate** could shut down the enzyme necessary for the production of glucose from lactic acid. Gold had chanced upon an **eminently logical way** of starving cancer. He immediately tested hydrazine sulfate on mice and found that in accord with his theory, the drug **inhibited both gluconeogenesis and tumor growth.**

Here is just one of many case studies of hydrazine sulfate's dramatic effects. In 1987, Erna Kamen, a sixty-three year old lung cancer patient, was administered hydrazine sulfate after her discharge from a Sarasota, Florida hospital. *"Basically, my mother was **sent home to die**,"* says Jeff Kamen, an Emmy-winning television reporter. *"She'd lost a significant amount of weight by then, and she had **no appetite** and virtually **no will to do anything**"* (eerily reminiscent of Marge's condition in 1994).

A doctor had told Jeff's father, Ira Kamen, that hydrazine sulfate offered at least **"a shot in the dark."** So one Monday in August 1987, a home nurse gave Mrs. Kamen **one hydrazine sulfate pill** shortly before serving lunch. *"On Tuesday morning,"* recalls Jeff, *"there was a commotion in the house. My mother had **risen from her bed** like the phoenix rising from the ashes. She was demanding that the nurse bring her downstairs so that she could* *have breakfast with me…When people you love get into this kind of facedown with death, you're just **incredibly grateful** for each moment."*

As Jeff describes his mother's recovery, *"her **searing pain was gone**; her appetite returned at a gallop."* Within three weeks, her racking cough had vanished and she could **walk unaided**. *"In the months before her death, she went on television with me to **tell the nation** about hydrazine sulfate. The National Cancer Institute stopped trashing hydrazine sulfate and began referring inquiries to the UCLA Medical School team whose work had **validated the effectiveness of the drug** long before Erna Kamen began taking it."* Jeff attributes his mother's death months later to her being *"mistakenly taken off hydrazine sulfate and subjected to an **unproven experimental substance**."*

With cancer patients, hydrazine sulfate is usually administered orally in 60-milligram capsules or tablets, approximately one to two hours before meals. It is given first once a day for several days, then twice a day, then three or four times daily, depending on the patient's response and the **physician's judgment**. On such a regimen, many terminal and semi-terminal patients have derived considerable benefit. Patients in the **early stages** of cancer derive the most benefit.

About half of the patients who get the drug administered in the early stages of cancer show an **almost immediate** weight gain and reversal of symptoms. In some instances, the tumor eventually disappears.

The common types of cancer most frequently reported to benefit from hydrazine sulfate therapy are recto-colon cancer, ovarian cancer, prostate cancer, lung cancer, Hodgkin's disease and other lymphomas, thyroid cancer, melanoma, and breast cancer.

These account for over **90 percent** of the cancers reported in this country.

Again, for further information on how to obtain this drug or research it further, do your own search on the Internet or look at Richard Walters book, *"Options."*

My Concerns

I do not recommend hydrazine sulfate as a self-treatment regimen because it does not have a proven safe dosage level and treatment regimen. You, of course, are free to form your own opinion. Certainly, it is cheap and readily available.

Immune Therapies

Long before Dr. Ghoneum discovered the natural substance he called MGN-3 in 1995, Big Pharma researchers had been working on ways to use the body's immune system to fight cancer. Right now, much of the research is centered on **vaccines**. You may hear about some of these, so it pays to be familiar with some of the terms.

Monoclonal antibodies are **synthetic cells** created through gene-splicing. The cancer patient's white blood cells are fused with his or her cancer cells. When the resulting *hybridomas* are reintroduced into the patient's body, they manufacture specific antibodies. These attack only cancer cells. Attached to anti-cancer drugs or natural toxins, **monoclonals serve as "guided missiles"** by directing the antibodies they manufacture toward their malignant prey.

Still in the research stage, monoclonals promise to be **tremendously expensive**. They will be a boon to the pharmaceutical-medical monopoly if they are ever used for cancer treatment. The media frequently touts them as the next cancer breakthrough.

The American Cancer Society freely admits that it will take *"many years to find the proper role of these [orthodox immunotherapy] agents in cancer treatment."* Knowledgeable observers say this means **another twenty years or more**. Meanwhile, the ACS continues to use its enormous power to **restrict or suppress** safe, non-toxic cancer therapies using immune system therapy that have produced **remarkable clinical results** in human beings. I cover several currently available immune system stimulants in Chapter 5. There were earlier natural immune therapies such as that of Lawrence Burton, Ph.D. (discussed below) and Virginia Livingston, M.D.

Coley's Mixed Bacterial Vaccine

Ironically, *Coley's mixed bacterial vaccine*, which has perhaps shown a greater cure rate than any other cancer treatment, is totally unavailable. Dr. William Coley (1862-1936) was an eminent New York City surgeon and Sloan-Kettering researcher. In the **1890s**, he developed a **vaccine** made of bacterial toxins that **activated immune-resistance mechanisms in cancer patients** and cured hundreds.

His daughter, Helen Coley Nauts, D.Sc., has preserved and carried forward his important work. Yet, despite the successful use of bacterial vaccines amply reported in the medical literature since the turn of the century, today's big drug companies have **no interest** in what they view as merely an **unprofitable** item.

The bottom line, dear readers, which is rather horrible to consider, is that at any one time, there are thousands of patients in the United States getting aggressive chemotherapy who would benefit from any immune-enhancing measures, even supportive nutrition or vitamin supplements. Do they get it? Unless they seek it out through publications like this one, the answer, sadly, is no.

Burton's Immuno-Augmentative Therapy

Dr. Lawrence Burton uses four blood proteins – substances occurring naturally in the body – to treat cancer. His Immuno-Augmentative Therapy (IAT), developed while he was a senior oncologist at St. Vincent's Hospital in New York City in the **1960s**, does not "attack" the cancer. Instead, it aims to **restore normal immune system functioning** so the patient's own immune system will destroy the cancer cells. Ask yourself what happened to the following evidence in the ensuing forty years.

Burton discovered that the components of the blood, which he called **blood fractions**, are deficient in the cancer patient. When they are present in correct balance, they work **synergistically** to control cancer cell growth and kill tumors.

His therapy involves replenishing the deficient blood fractions by injecting patients with them in amounts based on **daily or twice-daily blood analyses**. Patients continue to self-administer the injections from serum for whatever length of time is necessary, much like a diabetic takes insulin. IAT is **non-toxic and has no side effects.**

Dr. Burton does not claim that IAT is a cure. He describes it as a means to control and combat cancer. Yet, according to clinical records, **50 to 60%** of patients experience **tumor reduction**. Many undergo long-term regression. Some, even those with **terminal cancer**, have achieved **complete remission**.

Many cases of **metastatic cancer** of the colon and abdomen, treated with Burton's IAT, have gone well beyond five years of recovery. This is a remarkable achievement since the National Cancer Institute says these types of cancer have a **zero** five-year survival rate.

There is a clinic in the Bahamas treating patients today based on Burton's theory. For information on this clinic, go to:

http://www.immunemedicine.com

Cytoluminescent Therapy (CLT)

One of the newest wrinkles in cancer treatment is called "Cytoluminescent Therapy" (CLT). This has been known as Photodynamic Therapy (PDT), which was similar but used a different "sensitizing" agent. A clinic in Ireland specializes in CLT. Dr. Ralph Moss has visited them and published a report that was quite enthusiastic about the efficacy of this treatment. Recent rumors are that it is being introduced in the U.S.

I will quote for you an e-mail from a lady who visited the Ireland clinic for the treatment in late 2002. Here's how she described the treatment:

"…the theory behind CLT (PDT with a new agent) is that one ingests a sensitizing agent, this one is made from spirulina, which binds almost exclusively to cancer cells, and then infrared and LED light shined on the body will activate the agent through the blood (as it kind of rides to the cancer cells on the cholesterol-like substances in the blood), causing cellular excitement and creating singlet oxygen, an oxidative process, which in turn causes the cancer cells to basically blow up.

Lynnette"

Problems

In addition to the exorbitant cost ($20,000) and the fact that the Ireland clinic is booked for several months in advance, Lynette reports that they have been receiving many complaints about their lack of follow-up after the patient returns home – an essential part of this treatment. I have also heard that the original owners of the clinic had split up and were running competing clinics in Ireland.

The "Overnight Cancer Cure"

If you have read this far, I'd like to reward you with the description of a method of healing that not only has great promise, but has been used successfully on a few willing "guinea pigs" with advanced cancers. It has been dubbed the "Overnight Cancer Cure" (OCC).

This inexpensive and very effective treatment is described in detail at this web page:

http://www.New-Cancer-Treatments.org/Cancer/OCC.html

As the author of the web page, Webster Kehr, President of the Independent Cancer Research Foundation (see below), says:

"This cancer treatment is new. It is experimental, though it has been proven to be totally safe even for very advanced cancer patients. In other words, its safety is NOT experimental, only its effectiveness is experimental. This treatment is based heavily on a great deal of scientific evidence combined with solid cancer theory."

This treatment is so promising because it does not kill the cancer cells, causing all the "lysing" symptoms caused by "die-off" of the cancer cells. Instead, the "microbe" inside the cancer cell (viewed first by Royal Rife in the 1920's in his powerful microscope) is killed. The cancer cell then returns to normal cell operation, with the restoration of the "Krebs Cycle" (also called the "Citric Acid Cycle") and the "Electron Transport Chain" in the mitochondria.

The mitochondria are the molecules inside the cell which put out energy (also known as ATP) and control the apoptosis or cell death. They are inactive in the cancer cell. Once they can be reactivated (as they are with this treatment), the cell resumes the properties of cell death of a normal cell. The cancer cell then dies on its normal cycle – not as a cancer cell, but as if it was a normal cell. As such, it does not clog the liver, kidneys, lymph system and other organs with dead cancer cells, as most other cancer treatments do.

If you would like to understand the details of this treatment, which is backed up by hundreds of studies and several books on the subject, please read Webster's description of the treatment at the above web site. If you would like to read more about the theory of cancer, please go to:

http://www.New-Cancer-Treatments.org/Theory/CancerTheory.html

If all of this makes some sense to you, please consider a donation to the ICRF (see below) to help us with this important work.

"Natural Cancer Treatments That Work"

In March, 2003, an Australian team led by my friend Karon Beattie published the best set of reference books I have seen on "alternative" cancer treatments. This is actually four e-books. Karon updates them frequently. The price for this incredible collection of knowledge is unbelievable. Just $49.95. That's not for one, but all four of these great collections of information. The four books are:

Natural Cancer Treatments That Work

This is information on 350 different natural, non-toxic cancer treatments. It is 420 pages which include sources, web sites and history of each of these treatments. If you hear of a treatment that you think may work for you, I know of no better place to begin researching it.

I Beat Cancer

This e-book is a collection of 2,000 testimonials of people who healed their cancers using one or more of the treatments in the above book. It is cross-referenced by type of cancer and type of treatment.

How Successful Are Conventional Cancer Treatments?

This is an analysis of the studies of chemo, radiation and surgery. It is a great basis for you to arrive at true "informed consent" before you undergo one of these "therapies."

Who Can Help Me When I Have Cancer?

Here is help in finding caring people and organizations. There is information on financial support, doctor/clinic locators and many other worldwide resources.

Again, all four of these e-books are sold for just $49.95. Quite a bargain! To order them, just go to:

http://staywell.beatcancer.hop.clickbank.net

Cancer Success Forum

Karon Beattie, the principal author of the Natural Cancer Treatments e-books, has joined me in an effort to get you a place to get questions answered, post comments about your own treatment and, generally, communicate with other cancer patients. We call it the **Cancer Success Forum**. You will find it at:

http://www.CancerSuccessForum.com

Take a look at it. You need to read the brief "Rules." Then, click on the "Discussion Forum" link and see if there are any topics which interest you. If not, start a new topic. Someone -- Karon or me or some other Forum member -- will get you an answer.

I think you'll like this new way of communicating. Try it and see.

Lots of Cancer Therapies

The wide variety of cancer therapies that have proved effective over the past 50 years **boggles the mind**. I will simply list some more of them here to give you the words you need to research them further on the Internet or in Karon's e-books (above).

Asian herbs

Ayurveda

Bioelectric Therapies

Bovine Colustrum

Carctol

Chaparral

Chelation

Chinese Medicine

Chlorella

Co-enzyme Q10

Colloidal Silver

Concentrated Aloe Vera

Detoxification

DMSO Therapy

Far Infrared Therapy

Germanium

Gerson Therapy

Hans Nieper, M.D.

Haelan 951

Homeopathy

Hoxsey Therapy

Hyperbaric units

Hyperthermia

Immunocal

IP6

Issels' Whole-Body Therapy

Kelley's Nutritional-Metabolic Therapy

Lactoferrin

Live-Cell Therapy

Livingston Therapy

Lymphotonic PF2

Magnetic Sleep Pads

Mind-Body Treatments

Mistletoe (Iscador)

Moerman's Anti-Cancer Diet

MycoSoft

N-Tense

Noni Juice

Oncotox

Ozone Therapy

Psychotherapy

Peroxide Therapy

Rain-forest herbs

Selenium

T-Plus

Ukrain

VG-1000

Wigmore therapy

….and many more….
Check a few of those out on your favorite search engine. You'll
be amazed at the wealth of material on them. I have tried to
avoid information overload in this book by covering in detail the
treatments you should seriously consider. Obviously, this is a
judgment call. I am not dismissing any on the above list. Some
cancer patients have been healed by each of them.

Can You Help Us Help Others?

In July, 2008, the IRS finally approved the Independent Cancer
Research Foundation, Inc. (ICRF) to receive tax-dedutible
contributions. My four colleagues and I have been working on
this for about two years. Why did it take so long? Well, four of us
have business interests that are related to helping people heal
cancer. I, for example, sell this book and a coaching service for
cancer patients. Another member of our Board of Directors is an
M.D. with a practice. Another is an acupuncturist with a practice.
Another uses his VIBE Machine and other methods to help
people heal. We had to convince the IRS that we would not use
this foundation to promote our businesses. It took several
submissions to convince them that we are sincere. **We are.**

Please review the ICRF web site at:

http://www.New-Cancer-Treatments.org

What Will the Foundation Do?

People who come to the five members of the ICRF's Board of Directors tend to do so as a "last resort." All of us have wished for more proven remedies for "Stage IV" cancers. We are all convinced that with some research money we could perfect [and protect] certain cancer healing devices and substances that we feel are potentially effective for these "terminal" cancers where the person has been told by the doctor that "there is nothing more we can do." Some examples:

The Bob Beck Protocol

Bob Beck was an American inventor who played an important role in demonstrating the use of inexpensive electro-therapy machines. He invented a "Blood Purifier" and a "Magnetic Pulse Generator." He combined them with colloidal silver to heal cancer. Unfortunately, he did not live long enough after perfecting his inventions nor have enough financial backing to make his "protocol" widely available.

This is a proven protocol for healing advanced cancers. It just needs some **additional research** to establish its efficacy. Our plan, with really a small amount of money, is to fund research at a lab in Kansas which has agreed to work with us. Once the equipment and protocol are perfected, we will make it available to the public through a non-profit outlet.

The "Overnight Cancer Cure"

As I described above, Webster Kehr, President of the ICRF, has experimented with chlorine dioxide (also known as the **Miracle**

Mineral Supplement or MMS) mixed with dimethyl sulfoxide **(DMSO)**. Both of these substances have been used for many years to treat all kinds of degenerative conditions. The promise of this combination is very real. The ICRF Board Members and Jim Humble, the man who discovered MMS, are excited about the prospects of this mixture for treating advanced cancers.

A protocol has been worked out based on a few people willing to act as "guinea pigs" for us. What is needed now is **more testing** to perfect this protocol. We are quite sure that these two inexpensive substances hold the promise of a very effective healing regimen for **Stage IV cancers**. It will probably work best transdermally (through the skin). **Clinical testing is needed.** The ICRF can do this. All we need is some money (not very much!). Once this protocol is proven the mixture and instructions for its use can easily be **made available through non-profit outlets.**

These are just two examples of the types of work the ICRF will do. We need your help. None of the Board Members will be paid any compensation for work with the ICRF. They will be reimbursed for necessary travel. That's all.

How Can You Help?

The ICRF is now set up to **take your donations and account for their use**. Your donation is completely tax deductible on your 2008 and later year's Federal and State income tax return. Here are the details for donations:

Please make your checks out to **ICRF** and send them to:

Independent Cancer Research Foundation, Inc.
PO Box 2074
Lees Summit, MO 64063

The ICRF is tax-exempt under Section 501(c)(3) of the Internal Revenue Code and is classified as a "public charity." Your contributions to the ICRF are tax-deductible under Section 170 of the Code. The **Tax Identification number of the ICRF is 20-4461836.**

Who Are The Board of Directors?

The Board of Directors of the ICRF is composed of:

R. Webster Kehr, President and Chairman of the Board
System Administrator for Northrup Grumman for the past 6 years at Fort Leavenworth, Kansas. Worked for Sprint, also in Kansas, for the preceding 8 years. Part-time cancer researcher since 2001. Web site: http://www.CancerTutor.com.

Bill Henderson (me), Vice President and Secretary
Retired, living in California. Former Air Force officer (25 years) and publishing executive (18 years). Since 1998, has worked full-tme with cancer patients by phone and e-mail, published books and newsletters on "alternative" cancer healing, given workshops on "Beating Cancer – Gently." Since October, 2007, has hosted a weekly radio show called "How to Live Cancer-Free." Web sites: http://www.Beating-Cancer-Gently.com and http://www.WebTalkRadio.net.

Mike Vrentas, Vice President and Treasurer
Independent Insurance Agent in Missouri for Shelter Insurance Company. Former police officer in Kansas City, Missouri for 4 years. Part-time cancer researcher since 2002. Cherie, his wife, has summarized her cancer experience at: http://www.CheriesRoadToHealth.com.

Bill Wassall, M.D., Vice President
Medical Doctor – Radiologist in Louisiana. He provides advice to other members of the Board on medical issues and orthomolecular medicine. An expert on Vitamin C cancer research and treatment.

Gary Teal, Member of the Board
Board certified acupuncturist in private practice in Utah. An expert in electro-medicine.

Thank you for your generous contributions to help us with this life-saving work.

Conclusion

Do not trust the "system" to take care of your or your loved one's cancer. Get **proactive**. Do the research. Get knowledge. **Knowledge is power**.

Know this. Many different promising approaches to healing cancer and/or preventing its recurrence **now exist**.

You may want to travel to the Bahamas or Mexico or Germany or Spain but you don't have to any more. Your local health food store carries the things you need or you can order them from the sources I list in this book.

You may want to find a doctor who will help you use these treatments to augment "conventional" therapy and test your progress. You may want to **avoid conventional therapy completely**. Healing without any medical assistance is now **totally practical**. Do your own healing and testing, if you feel comfortable with it. If not, at least **start on the self-treatment regimen** while you look for that perfect doctor. There is one out there. I would never choose an oncologist, radiologist or cancer surgeon. Your choice may be different from mine, but **keep looking**. I know of competent cancer doctors who use gentle, non-toxic healing techniques in the United States, Canada, Mexico, Singapore, Malaysia, Great Britain, Germany, South America and most other countries. Use the Directories I provided in Chapter 1 of this book.

Don't Wait For More Proof

Many of these "alternative" therapies are **urgently** in need of more research to bring out their full potential. You can make this happen sooner by supporting our ICRF.

Dr. Robert C. Atkins, who many of you may know because of his nutrition books, put it quite succinctly. He said:

*"There have been **many** cancer cures, and all have been ruthlessly and systematically suppressed with a Gestapo-like thoroughness by the cancer establishment. The cancer establishment is the not-too-shadowy association of the American Cancer Society, the leading cancer hospitals, the National Cancer Institute, and the FDA. The shadowy part is the fact that these respected institutions are very much dominated by members and friends of members of the pharmaceutical industry, which profits so incredibly much from our profession-wide obsession with chemotherapy."*

It is hard for most Americans to believe that life-saving and valid therapies are being **suppressed deliberately**. It just doesn't seem possible in modern America. Unfortunately, most Americans are **dead wrong**. The cancer establishment has an **eighty-year history** of corruption, incompetence, and **deliberate suppression** of cancer therapies that actually work. This includes the rigging of clinical trials at major institutions in order to **discredit non-toxic, natural therapies**. Barry Lynes has documented this well in his book *The Healing of Cancer* as has Daniel Haley in *Politics In Healing*. See Appendix A for more information on these books. As Lynes says, *"The American Cancer Society is not interested in a cure. It would go out of business."*

Cancer Research Is Fraud

Two-time Nobel laureate Linus Pauling summed up the situation well when he said, *"Everyone should know that the 'war on cancer' is largely a **fraud**, and that the National Cancer Institute and the American Cancer Society are **derelict in their duties** to the people who support them."*

According to Barry Lynes, *"At a minimum, the American Cancer Society…should be investigated by the U. S. Justice Department for **fraud**, false advertising, **conspiracy** and a variety of other anti-trust, monopolistic crimes."*

Closely linked to the ACS through interlocking directorates is the National Cancer Institute. Funded by the government, and founded in 1937 this agency currently has a budget of over 4 **billion dollars a year**. Wouldn't you expect such an agency to be a catalyst for **innovation**? Shouldn't they openly encourage any new technique or method that might slow the death count in the **cancer epidemic** that claims 10,000 American lives every week?

NCI is **just the opposite**. It is a repressive guardian of the status quo that funds an **"old boys' network"** committed to chemotherapy and radiation. They actively conspire with other government agencies to **harass or thwart** innovative alternative cancer therapies.

Instead of serving the public, *"NCI created a bureaucratic haven for scientism, filled with **committee procedures**, payoffs, **collusion with drug companies** and **interminable roadblocks** for the truly innovative cancer fighters,"* as Barry Lynes observes in *The Healing of Cancer*.

What the NCI does with their $4 billion in taxes each year is a unique form of **corruption** in the history of science. NCI distributes these billions in research grants and, together with the ACS, sets the dominant trends in research. Incredibly, **90 % of the members** of NCI's peer review committee get NCI money for **their own research**. **70% of ACS's research budget** goes to individuals or institutions with which the ACS board members are **personally affiliated.**

*"In any other part of government, it would be a **corrupt practice** for the persons giving out the money and the persons getting it to be the same people,"* says Irwin Bross, Ph.D., former Director of Biostatistics at the famed Roswell Park Memorial Institute, the nation's oldest cancer research hospital. Testifying before a congressional subcommittee, Dr. Bross added, *"It is a corrupt practice even when it is called 'peer review' or 'cancer research'...This set-up is not worth revamping and should **simply be junked."***

Don't Be A Statistic

You need look no further than the **statistics on cancer deaths**. The death rates from the six major killer cancers – cancers of the lung, colon, breast, prostate, pancreas, and ovary – have either stayed the same or increased during the past **sixty years**. If this is a "war on cancer" it has **long since been lost**.

Unlike many other countries, the United States supports only **one kind of medicine**. Because of this, Americans have been denied many vital aspects of the **science and art of healing**. *"Your family doctor is no longer free to choose the treatment he or she feels is best for you, but must follow the dictates established by physicians whose motives and alliances are such that their decisions may not be in your best interests,"* says Alan Levin, M.D.

Your Right Of Choice

Patients' most fundamental right – **medical freedom of choice** – has been lost in this country. The medical monopoly's **right to make money** comes before your right to decide – in consultation with your doctor – which cancer therapy would be **best** for your particular condition. The following letter eloquently and movingly illustrates the **dilemma faced** by the cancer patient. The author is a psychologist.

"My wife was diagnosed as having terminal ovarian cancer five years ago. She is alive, well and healthy because of non-approved and unconventional cancer treatment.

I am writing this as a letter of protest and in an attempt to educate you and possibly save your life or that of your wife or child. I am not a crazy fanatic, but I am a 48-year-old man who, five years ago, had to decide what to do in order to try to save my wife's life. We investigated and researched our options and made an informed and intelligent decision to seek something other than what was offered by traditional medicine in this country.

I am angry, frustrated, and mad as hell that I have had to take my wife out of this country, had to struggle with my health insurance company because her treatment was 'not approved,' and had to struggle to obtain her medications because they are 'not approved' and subject to confiscation. It has been a battle to provide her with alternative cancer treatment.

I now know that there is a financial war going on, and the victims are the millions of people who have been denied alternative cancer treatments because the AMA or FDA or someone has decided that we can only undergo an approved treatment…There are no rights to life or liberty in this country when it comes to freedom of choice in medicine. There is only coercion and subversion and greed – and people dying. We are the financial prisoners of the AMA and FDA, and they are killing us in the name of approved treatment.

My wife was almost a victim; and if you allow this to continue, then one day you will become a victim, too.

Please help to do something to bring truth, sanity and morality back to health care in America."

Live Long and Die Young!

Thank you for reading this book. Please read the booklets on **prevention** and **treatment** of cancer and other degenerative disease with proper **diet and exercise**. Let's avoid becoming victims.

If you or a relative or friend suffers from either a **sore back** or **diabetes**, please read those booklets, also.

If you already are engaged in the battle of survival with cancer, I sincerely hope that I have given you **ammunition and hope**.

May God Bless You with a long and healthy life!!

Bill Henderson
Author, "Cure Your Cancer" and "Cancer-Free"
Web site: http://www.Beating-Cancer-Gently.com
E-mail: uhealcancer@gmail.com
Weekly radio show: http://www.WebTalkRadio.net
"How to Live Cancer-Free"
Listen anytime.

APPENDIX A
RESOURCE
SUMMARY

Following is a summary of the sources mentioned in this book and some others of interest. To get to the websites mentioned, simply click on the underlined link (if you're reading this on your computer). Your web browser will open and take you to the website. When you close your browser, you'll come back to the same place in this book. If you're reading this in a paperback book, you'll have to type the web site addresses in your browser window.

1. *REAL AGE – Are You As Young As You Can Be?*, *b*y Michael F. Roizen, M.D. , copyright 1999. Website: http://www.realage.com

Learn how each part of your lifestyle affects your lifespan. Is your "Real Age" older or younger than what's on your driver's license? Once you take the test, you will have perfect knowledge of what changes in your lifestyle will be the most beneficial. At the website, you can also subscribe to a free e-mail service that will deliver daily tips on improving your health and longevity to your e-mail box.

2. *Antioxidants Against Cancer* by Ralph W. Moss, PhD, copyright 2000. Website: http://CancerDecisions.com

This book should be "required reading" for everyone, not just cancer patients. All of us need to be familiar with the antioxidants. This book has lots of detail about specific compounds and their effects on different types of cancer. Many of them have an anti-cancer effect as well. At his web site, you will be able to order any of his 10 books on cancer plus a 400+ page report on each of over 210 cancer diagnoses. These cover both conventional and alternative treatments; supplements you should take, or avoid; and information on European and Mexican clinics. A monthly telephone or e-mail update on each report is also available.

3. *Alternatives* newsletter by David G. Williams, M.D. Website: http://www.DrDavidWilliams.com

Dr. Williams is quoted extensively in this book. For over 20 years, he has traveled the world in search of the best cures for all common diseases. His website has a complete catalog of his newsletters, organized by subject. You can read a synopsis of each article and order those that interest you. I have subscribed to his newsletter since 1985. I have found no better source for a wide variety of health information.

4. *Questioning Chemotherapy*, by Ralph W. Moss, PhD, copyright 1995. Website: http://www.CancerDecisions.com

A complete discussion of the limitations of chemotherapy for the treatment of cancer. If you or a loved one or friend have cancer, you must read this book. It gives you detailed information on each medication used and how effective it is for each type of cancer. Do not agree to any chemotherapy treatment until you read this book cover to cover.

5. *World Without Cancer – The Story of Vitamin B17*, by G. Edward Griffin, copyright 1997 and 1974 –

Fifteenth printing: March 2000. Available at Amazon.com.

The first half of this book presents a detailed and documented history of Laetrile (Vitamin B17) and its use in cancer treatment. It describes in detail the suppression of this compound by the Food and Drug Administration (FDA) and the "cyanide scare" used to justify it. The second half covers "The Politics of Cancer Therapy." The author describes a conspiracy involving American moguls, Nazi officers in Hitler's Germany and the drug industry in general. Fasten your seat belt. This is a very well-written but controversial book. There are several reader reviews available at Amazon.com. For more information on Laetrile/amygdalin/Vitamin B17, see Chapter 7 above.

6. *The Healing of Cancer*, by Barry Lynes, copyright 1989 distributed in the United States by Vitamart, K-Mart Plaza, Route 10, Randolph, NJ 08869; (201) 366-4494.

A hard-hitting expose of the medical establishment's fifty-year history of suppressing alternative cancer therapies. American journalist Barry Lynes discusses various alternative treatments in this incisive analysis.

7. *Resonant Frequency Therapy – Building the Rife Beam Ray Device*, by James E. Bare, D.C., copyright 1995.

If you are interested, you can purchase the book. The book includes detailed instructions for building the Beam Ray Device. My personal opinion is that this device has been made obsolete by several of the natural cancer therapies discussed in this book and by the VIBE Machine.

8. *The Cure For All Cancers*, by Hulda Regehr Clark, PhD, , N.D., copyright 1993.

This book documents Dr. Clark's treatment of over 100 cancer cases. She uses an electronic device to isolate the cancer sites. The instructions for building it are in the book. Her theory on the cause of cancer by parasites or intestinal flukes is not completely original. It is interesting and controversial.

For more information on Dr. Clark, go to the web site: http://www.drclark.ch

9. *Creating Health – How to Wake Up The Body's Intelligence*, by Deepak Chopra, M.D., copyright 1987. Website: http://www.chopra.com

This is Dr. Chopra's "breakthrough" book – the first in which he created a new understanding of health and illness and the healing power of the mind. He has since written over 25 books, translated into 35 languages, plus over 100 audio and videotape series. In 1999, Time Magazine selected Dr. Chopra as one of the "Top 100 Icons and Heroes of The Century." You will understand his later work better if you read this book first. His theories about mind-body interaction have now been proven. The scientific proof is covered in the next book on this list.

10. *The Balance Within – The Science Connecting Health and Emotions*, by Esther M. Sternberg, M.D., copyright 2000.

Dr. Sternberg is a leading expert on the interaction of the endocrine and immune systems, with impressive credentials. She takes us from the origins of medicine in Greece, to the early medical schools in Padua, to modern research in

Montreal and the U.S. She clearly describes how we came to appreciate the physiology of stress, how the mind influences the body, and how the body affects the mind. This area of research, in which Dr. Sternberg has been one of the world's leading scientists for at least a decade, is leading to new understandings and treatments of the stress-related diseases of modern life.

> 11. American Holistic Health Association, P. O. Box 17400, Anaheim, CA 92817. Phone: (714) 779-6152. Website: http://healthy.net/ahha

At this website, you can enter search criteria (zip code, telephone area code, state, specialty, etc.) and get a list of "holistic" doctors with their specialties in your area.

> 12. American Holistic Medical Association, 6728 Old McLean Village Drive, McLean, VA 22101. Phone: (703) 556-9728 FAX: (703) 556-8729. Website: http://www.holisticmedicine.org/

At this website, you will find information about this group. If you want a directory of their members, you will need to send them $10.

> 13. The Simonton Cancer Center, P. O. Box 890, Pacific Palisades, CA 90272. Toll free: (800) 459-3424; Local: (310) 457-3811; FAX: (310) 457-0421. E-mail: simonton@lainet.com. Website: http://www.simontoncenter.com/

Dr. Simonton is famous for pioneering studies in the use of the mind to overcome cancer and other diseases. You may also want to read his book *Getting Well Again*. It covers the mental processes essential in recovering from advanced and terminal cancer and other serious ailments.

14. WebMD Health. Website: http://my.webmd.com

A **very** comprehensive website covering all aspects of health care – conventional and alternative/complementary. This website is a perfect example of the information available through the Internet. Search capability, chat rooms, research results, etc. All-encompassing and **complete**. It is also an example of one of the **main reasons I wrote this book**. Laymen need a guide to the vast amount of information available. Without that, it can be **overwhelming**.

15. American Diabetes Association. Website: http://diabetes.org

Another comprehensive website for diabetes sufferers. It covers both Type 1 and Type 2 diabetes. Emphasis is on **diet and exercise**. If you have diabetes or suspect you have it, **go here**. Same comments about comprehensive nature of this site as those for WebMD Health above.

16. *The Complete Encyclopedia of Natural Healing*, by Gary Null, September, 2000.

Gary Null has been updating this reference book since it was first published in 1988. It is written for the layperson but written by an expert. The listings are by ailment, so you can look under whatever ails you – asthma, heart disease, arthritis, diabetes, allergies, cancer, etc. – and take whatever vitamins or herbs are helpful for that specific condition. This book is also available from amazon.com. The last time I checked, it was $16.

17. *An Alternative Medicine Definitive Guide to Cancer* by W. John Diamond, W. Lee Cowden and Burton Goldberg, March, 1997.

This massive (1,116 pages) book is published by the editors of the magazine *Alternative Medicine*. The first section consists of richly detailed accounts of the successful cancer treatment plans of 23 respected alternative physicians from Robert C. Atkins to Charles B. Simone. Part 2 is a fundamental explanation of the nature, causes, politics and prevention of cancer. The final section presents alternative therapies from a to z. It is meant for those who have cancer, their friends and family and (who knows?) maybe even their doctor! It is also available from amazon.com for $49.95. They have used ones available for $29.95. I recently discovered a slimmed down version of this hefty tome. It is called *Cancer Diagnosis – What to Do Next* by the same authors. Only $14.95.

18. *Racketeering in Medicine: The Suppression of Alternatives*, by James P. Carter, September 1992.

Carter describes in detail how, for years, the AMA, FDA and pharmaceutical industry have tried to discredit alternative, less expensive, less invasive and often more effective methods of treatment. He does not sensationalize the topic but documents with evidence how the governing bodies of modern medicine have a vested interest in suppressing these treatments and making sure that average folks never know about them. If you have any doubts about this after reading my book, get James Carter's. If he doesn't convince you, I doubt that anything will. This one, too, is available from amazon.com, price: $10.36, with used ones for $7.95.

19. *Options – The Alternative Cancer Therapy Book*, by Richard Walters, copyright 1993, published by Avery.

A comprehensive guide to all forms of alternative cancer therapy known at the time this book was published (1993). Walters has thoroughly documented 28 such therapies. In much more detail than I can do here, he lays out the case that suppression of valid cancer therapies has been a common practice of the American cancer "establishment" for at least the last 50 years.

20. Lorraine Day, M.D. Website: http://www.drday.com

Dr. Day is an orthopedic surgeon. She spent 15 years on the faculty at the University of California at San Francisco School of Medicine. She was also the Chief of Orthopedic Surgery at San Francisco General Hospital.

At her website, you'll be able to purchase a video of her describing how she cured herself of metastasized breast cancer. There are remarkable photos of her **grapefruit-sized tumor** protruding from her chest. Many of her videos on cancer can be purchased at her website. The video titles will give you an idea of her **wonderful healing message**:

"Cancer Doesn't Scare Me Anymore"
"Drugs Never Cure Disease"
"Diseases Don't Just Happen"
and
"Sorting Through The Maze Of Alternative Medicine"

Don't miss this website.

21. Moderated chat room. http://aoma.com/cs

The "cs" in the site name stands for "cancer survivors." This is a "real time" chat room. They are merging with "OncoChat," another chat room for cancer survivors. Here you will find others with an interest in cancer therapy. The advantage of a moderated chat room is that you usually get a relatively "instant" answer to your question.

22. *A Dietician's Cancer Story*, by Diana Dyer.

This lady self-published her 54-page cancer and nutrition booklet in 1997. It was once a best-selling cancer and nutrition book on amazon.com. She has set up an endowment with proceeds from the booklet to help underwrite research about how good nutrition can prevent the recurrence of cancer. For more information, go to:

http://www.DianaDyerMSRD.com

23. The Cancer Cure Foundation

Once you have read my book, you need to explore this company's site. It is a non-profit organization dedicated to providing information on alternative cancer therapies. At their web site, you will find detailed descriptions of multiple clinics all over the world. They are divided into "Clinics in the U.S.," "Clinics in Mexico," and "Clinics Outside the U.S. and Mexico." They include contact names, phone numbers, addresses, web sites, e-mail addresses, pictures of providers, pictures of the clinics, and pictures of patients with their testimonials. They give a detailed description of the type of treatment given by each clinic, including glossaries of terms. Finally, they give you a list of 8 or 10 of the "Most Popular" clinics. They ask for feedback from their users and obviously they get it. They have been doing this since 1976, but they have adapted their service very efficiently to the Internet Age. Go to:

http://cancure.org

24. Annie Appleseed Project

An awesome lady. Ann Fonfa has taken up the torch for all cancer patients in a very courageous and vivacious way. You need to get to know this lady. At her web site, among dozens of other resources, you will be able to read her three-week diary kept during her successful treatment for breast cancer at the Gerson Clinic in Tijuana, Mexico. She lobbies constantly for more research into Complementary & Alternative Medicine (CAM). She is championing your interests. Don't miss this site:

http://www.AnnieAppleseedProject.org

25. Dr. Ron Kennedy's web site.

This wonderful doctor's web site contains an encyclopedic summary of all the alternative treatments. There is even a search engine where you can enter your Zip Code and get a list of doctors or dentists in one or more of the "alternative" specialties in your area of the country.

http://www.medical-library.net/sites/adjunctive_therapies_for_cancer.html

26. Dr. Matthias Rath's web site

This outstanding German doctor has a very educational pdf booklet on the nature of cancer and its metastasis. Don't miss this one!

http://www4.dr-rath-foundation.org/pdf-files/cancerresearch.pdf

27. Insulin Potentiation Therapy (IPT).

If you have cancer, you need to consider this form of low-dose chemotherapy. Side effects are minimal and the effects of the chemo are magnified several thousand times by using an insulin shot 30 minutes or so before administering the chemo drug (in a very weak dose). This web site includes a

list of all the physicians (about 108 at this writing) who are
qualified in this important therapy.

http://iptforcancer.com

Other web sites with lots of information on IPT are:

http://iptq.com

http://ElkaBest.com

  28. Art Brown's web site.

Art Brown has written a book similar to mine. He is an active
participant in several on-line forums concerning cancer
treatments. Art is a former employee of the Cancer Cure
Foundation. His web site is:

http://www.alternative-cancer.net

  29. National Cancer Research Foundation

At Fred Eichhorn's interesting web site, you'll find lots of
testimonials from cancer survivors – all types of cancer. Fred
works hard and charges little to help heal lots of cancer
patients. His web site is:

http://www.ncrf.org

  30. CancerEducation.com

One of the best sites for comprehensive cancer information.
You can see lectures by famous cancer experts. One
example: A 71-minute slide show and lecture by Dr. William
Fair. Dr. Fair has been on the staff of Memorial Sloan-
Kettering Cancer Center in New York for 18 years as a

urologist. He was diagnosed with colon cancer in the early 90's. After two bouts with chemo, and two recurrences, he cured himself with "alternative" methods and has become a zealot about informing people about the inadequacy of the cancer treatments in the allopathic (conventional) medicine system.

http://www.CancerEducation.com

31. Life Extension Foundation

One of the best sources for information about prevention of all degenerative disease, including cancer. They publish a monthly magazine and (of course) a line of supplements. Their prices don't come close to Our Health Coop, so use this as an information source only.

http://www.lef.org

32. *Beating Cancer With Nutrition* by Patrick Quillin, copyright 2001.

A useful book for cancer patients to understand their diet choices and a slew of great recipes to help you implement them. One caution: Pat Quillin has not heard of the Budwig cottage cheese/flaxseed oil diet (see Chapter 5).

33. *The pH Miracle* by Dr. Robert Young, copyright 2002.

Here is the ultimate logic behind your body's need to alkalize to stay healthy.

34. *10 Natural Remedies That Can Save Your Life*, by James Balch, M.D., copyright 2000.

Dr. Balch discusses enzymes and other natural treatments in detail. $19 in paparback from amazon.com. Also available in an audio playback download for $12.95.

    35. *Lessons From The Miracle Doctors*, by Jon Barron, copyright 2002.

A 169-page PDF download e-book (like this one) that is chock full of information on getting and staying well. Covers all types of illness from the CAM viewpoint.

    36. *Saving Yourself from the Disease-Care Crisis*, by Walt Stoll, M.D., copyright 1996.

A treatise on coping with common ailments and the effects of stress on your health.

    37. *Alive And Well – One Doctor's Experience With Nutrition in the Treatment of Cancer Patients*, by Philip E. Binzel, M.D.

An intriguing account of this conventional doctor's epiphany about the importance of nutrition in the healing of cancer.

    38. Gavin Phillips web site.

Gavin is a dedicated crusader for alternative cancer cures. His non-profit web site: http://www.cancerinform.org has a wealth of background information for you on why we all need to co-doctor. First, you need to read the article he wrote which was published in "Clamor" magazine in 2001.

http://www.cancerinform.org/article.html

Browse Gavin's web site. You'll be impressed, as I was, at both his knowledge and his sincerity in fighting for your right to medical choice.

39. Alkalize for Health web site.

The web site "Alkalize for Health" is a comprehensive site. Among other things, it features a recipe for "Cancer Self-Treatment." You can find it at:

http://www.alkalizeforhealth.net/cancerselftreatment.htm

The eight-part program they outline for curing or preventing cancer includes information on: Cancer and Oxygen; The Importance of Exercise; Cancer and Ph; Acidity and Free Radicals; Purification Techniques; Enzymes to Dissolve Cancers; Vitamins to Fight Cancer; and Cancer and Meditation.

When you finish reading those 17 pages, you'll understand cancer a lot better. Check out their more in depth coverage of oxygen, alkalinity, meditation and hyperthermia. If you are more comfortable with another language, this site can be read in French, German, Italian, Portugese and Spanish.

40. CancerCured online forum.

If you are interested in joining the discussion forum on Yahoo Groups from which I get lots of my information, just send a blank e-mail to:

mailto:cancercured-subscribe@yahoogroups.com

You can just monitor the messages from well-informed people like Art Brown if you don't feel like contributing.

41. Direct Labs – do-it-yourself blood tests.

There is a new (at least new to me) service available now in the U.S. You can obtain your own blood tests, including some cancer tests, without going through your doctor for a "prescription" for the lab.

Take a look at this web site:

http://www.directlabs.com/

When you call them, they will direct you to a local blood lab in your area for getting a sample drawn. The lab will perform the tests and then mail the results in plain English directly to you. If you prefer, you can have the results sent to a doctor.

42. Natural Solutions Foundation

Since 2004, Dr. Rima Laibow and Major General Albert Stubblebine III (US Army, Retired) have traveled the world touting freedom of choice in health care. They have convinced several governments to support them in their fight against the spread of the limitations on natural supplements imposed by the EU in European countries. Called "Codex Alimentarius," this ridiculous limitation on the supplements you use may come to the U.S. soon. To help them avoid this, please contribute to their effort at:

http://www.HealthFreedomUSA.org

43. "Cancer – Step Outside The Box" by Ty Bollinger

After losing seven of his family members to conventional cancer treatment, Ty Bollinger decided to do something about this horrible scourge. He has. His book, "Cancer -- Step Outside The Box," published in 2006, is remarkable in its thorough discussion of both the "disease" (I prefer to call it a "reaction") and its treatment.

If you want complete information on cancer, Ty's book is the place to look. Please don't be put off by Ty's incorporation of his sincere religious beliefs in his writing. This book is priceless to the cancer patient as an information source, including a chapter called "The Top Five Stage IV Treatments" and another called "The Overnight Cancer Cure (O.C.C.)." There is a great Appendix on "Recommended Cancer Clinics" and a Glossary and Index. This is a very professional job at compiling all the current information on alternative cancer treatment. Buy it. This young man deserves to be rewarded for a magnificent effort to inform cancer patients. You can order it at amazon.com or bn.com.

44. "Reverse Aging" by Sang Whang

Want to extend your life? Mr. Whang has told you how in this book. It's as simple as drinking "ionized" water with its high alkalinity. This is the most complete and convincing description of this science I have seen. Get it, as I did, at amazon.com. To see one of the water filters he is discussing, and my wife and I are using, just go to:

http://www.BetterWayHealth.com

45. Raymond Francis and The Project to End Disease (TPED)

I recently interviewed Raymond Francis on my web talk radio show. He has a world-wide movement underway called "The Project to End Disease." For details on how you can help, please go to *http://www.TPED.org*. Raymond's own web site is: *http://www.BeyondHealth.com*.

Booklet #1 – Stop Your Aging With Diet

Someday we will sit down to a banquet of our own consequences.
Robert Louis Stevenson

A HEALTHY DIET

All of us have read about **diets**. Most of us have tried one or more. Most of them have been **unsuccessful** in terms of long-term benefit. Why?

Diets are seen as **temporary**. "I'll get on this diet and lose 20 pounds." Then what? To be **healthy forever**, you must simply adopt **eating habits** that are healthy. Nothing else works. If you don't believe me, ask your friends. Ask them to tell you about a diet where they **permanently** lost xx pounds. Do your own survey.

For now, let's assume that **no diet** is worth the paper it is written on. **Healthy eating habits** are what we're talking about. Here are two books – culled from the dozens of nutrition and dietary books I've read – which will help you the most.DI

"DIET WISE"

We want to eat healthy. **Forever**. What does that involve? I gave you my advice for cancer patients in Chapter 5. That approach works for healthy people, too. There is one more concern which you need to be aware of. **Food allergies.**

261

Advice from a Real Expert

One of the more interesting people I have interviewed on my web talk radio show is **Dr. Keith Scott-Mumby**, . A fully qualified M.D. in Great Britain for 27 years, Dr. Keith moved to the U.S. several years ago. In Great Britain, his specialty was food allergies. He has treated thousands of patients, helped them discover their food allergies and renewed their lives. Beginning in 1985, he has written **five books** on the subject.

In his latest book, *"Diet Wise – Let Your Body Choose The Food That's Right For You"* published in 2007, Dr. Scott-Mumby has consolidated all his experience in **one great book**. Just a couple of examples of his experience with his patients from this book should convince you to read it.

One of his patients had been suffering from chronic health problems for 20 years. She felt she ate a healthy diet with **lots of vegetables.** Once Dr. Keith convinced her to try his **"elimination and challenge diet"** procedure, she found she was **allergic to lettuce!** Once the lettuce was eliminated from her diet, she lost all her symptoms within a couple of weeks.

Another of his patients had found she was **allergic to potatoes**. She thought she had eliminated them completely but some of her symptoms continued. Some detective work found that the **Vitamin B6 tablets** she was taking daily contained potatoes as **part of the "binder"** in the pill. Once she stopped taking those pills, she lost all her symptoms almost immediately.

Dr. Keith is quite convinced, after his experience with **thousands of patients**, that all of us have allergic reactions to at least one type of food. Some of us react to **eight or nine different types** of food. Reactions can be triggered by tiny doses.

In "Diet Wise," he lists the **"top ten"** foods, one or more of which cause allergic reactions in most of us. They are: **wheat, corn, egg, milk, tea, coffee, cane sugar, yeast, citrus fruit (usually orange) and cheese.**

With lots of convincing examples like those above, I'm quite sure you will want to try his elimination and challenge diet. He explains the procedure **in great detail.** Once you have eliminated all the usual suspects for five days, the "challenge" phase nails for you **the food which has been causing your physical problems**.

Just the titles of a few chapters from this great book will, I hope, convince you that this book is a **must** for you to read. Here are several chapter headings:

The Myths of Nutritional Medicine
The Hidden, or "Masking Effect" Explained
Overload and Target Organs
Brain Allergies
Self Inventory
What to do if the Diet Succeeds
What to do if the Diet Fails
Problem Situations You May Encounter in Elimination Dieting
Disordered Glucose Metabolism (Hypoglycemia)
Malabsorption and leaky gut
Candida, yeast and mold

There is much more in this book, including five Appendices with useful recipes, addresses of helpful agencies and reference material.

How to Get This Book

Here are four web sites which will give you much more information compiled by Dr. Keith Scott-Mumby and where you can buy his *"Diet Wise"* book.

http://www.DietWiseBook.com

and

http://www.Alternative-Doctor.com

and

http://www.Alternative-Doctor-Radio.com

and

http://Healing-Devices.com

You'll find a **wealth of information** at these sites, including a **free e-book** at the first one and **teleseminars and newsletters** at the second one. If you want to get educated on the real causes of your physical problems and how to heal them – or avoid them – you'll find **no better information source anywhere**.

"THE CHINA STUDY"

When I first read the book *"The China Study"* by T. Colin Campbell, PhD, I thought **"Wow, finally a nutrition book based on science."** The dozens of nutrition and dietary books I had read up to then were **almost all opinion**. They differed radically in their suggestions and disagreed on basic principles. Even within these books were contradictions. This book is **radically different.**

Dr. Campbell is a professor on nutrition at Cornell University. For more than forty years, he has been at the forefront of nutrition research. His legacy, *"The China Study,"* is the most comprehensive study of health and nutrition ever conducted. This book was the culmination of a twenty-year partnership of Cornell University, Oxford University and the Chinese Academy of Preventive Medicine.

Don't let the fact that this book is **"peer-reviewed science"** turn you off. It is written in a **very readable style**. The difference from other books of this type is that all of Dr. Campbell's conclusions are **backed up with statistical data**. Much of it was drawn from a ten-year study he conducted in China and Taiwan. Over **8,000 people in 65 counties** were involved in this study. Meticulous records were kept of **what they ate and the resulting health status**. This study is just one of the many scientific studies used for the conclusions in this book.

Dr. Campbell's chapter on *"Turning Off Cancer"* alone should make you very happy to have bought and read this **very useful book.** So, what are his conclusions? The principal one is that the **people who ate the least animal protein were the healthiest.** If you want a summary of his conclusions, it is these four words: **"whole food – plant based."**

Among other useful information for cancer patients, you will discover that cancer can be **"turned on" and "turned off"** by simply adjusting your intake of **dairy products** and **other animal protein**. As he points out, laboratory studies have shown that **both these common parts of the American diet cause cancer**. By eliminating them, cancer heals.

After reading this book, my wife and I have limited our intake of animal protein (meat, fish, shellfish, chicken, turkey, eggs, etc.) to **one helping a week.** We had already eliminated dairy products.

Not convinced? Just read the book and study the statistics. Dr. Campbell proves **beyond doubt** that these two sources of protein – along with sugar and processed food – are the **major causes of the cancer epidemic** in so-called "civilized" nations.

This book, published in 2006, is easily available at Amazon.com and in most book stores. I **strongly recommend** you read it to reinforce your commitment to **drastically and permanently** change your diet to overcome or prevent cancer (and all other degenerative conditions).

A HEALTHY MIND

Recent discoveries **prove** the thesis that there is a real **"mind-body connection."** We will discuss these below. **Deepak Chopra, M.D.** was the first author to make this connection clear to me.

Meet Dr. Chopra

Dr. Chopra has now written **25 books** that have been translated into **35 languages**. He has produced **over 100** audio and videotape series. In 1999, Time magazine selected Dr. Chopra as one of the **"Top 100 Icons and Heroes of the Century."**

I first encountered Dr. Chopra in his book called *Creating Health* in 1990 or so. Shortly after reading that book, my wife, Marge and I ordered a set of audiotapes he made called *"Ageless Body, Timeless Mind."* I have found him to be an excellent source for wisdom on the **interconnections** between physical, mental, emotional and spiritual health.

I cannot improve on his words, so I will quote them from his book *"Creating Health:"*

"How to Be Perfectly Healthy and Feel Ever Youthful

HEALTH IS OUR NATURAL STATE. The World Health Organization has defined it as something more than the absence of disease or infirmity -- health is the state of perfect physical, mental, and social well-being. To this may be added spiritual well-being, a zest for life, a sense of fulfillment, and an awareness of harmony with the universe around him. It is a state in which one feels ever youthful, ever buoyant, and ever happy. Such a state is not only desirable but also quite possible. And it is not only quite possible, it is easy to obtain."

As an experienced **medical doctor**, Chopra saw the limitations of "conventional" medicine. The **certainty** of the connection between emotions, attitudes, spiritual awareness and physical health arose from his **clinical practice**. This "epiphany" of the **"mind-body connection"** occurred to him over 20 years ago...in the mid '80s. He has devoted his life since then to bringing this message to people using all forms of media.

To understand and appreciate his message, you really need to **read one or more** of his early works. All available from **amazon.com**, they include:

Creating Health -- How to Wake Up the Body's Intelligence, originally published in 1987, most recent revision in September 1995.

Quantum Healing -- Exploring the Frontiers of Mind/Body Medicine, originally published in August 1991,

Perfect Health -- The Complete Mind/Body Guide, originally published in August 1991.

Because his work covers a **complete view** of the universe and everything in it, it is **presumptuous** to quote **excerpts**. Let me instead quote a "blurb" from the jacket of *"Creating Health."* Hopefully, this will **pique your interest** to get at least this one book and enjoy it.

"Creating Health was a breakthrough book -- the first in which Deepak Chopra created a new understanding of health and illness and the healing power of the mind.

Dr. Chopra is considered the preeminent spokesman for the six-thousand-year-old tradition of health care from India -- Ayurveda. In this book he blends Eastern and Western medical philosophy for a clearer, richer view of the road to perfect health, a balance between mind, body, and spirit.

An endocrinologist, Dr. Chopra has practiced in the Boston area since 1971 and is former chief of staff of New England Memorial Hospital in Stoneham, Massachusetts. He is now medical director of the Maharishi Ayurveda Health Center for Stress Management and Behavioral Medicine in Lancaster, Massachusetts."

Scientific Proof

In just the last few years, researchers in a **variety of fields** have concluded that the ideas expressed by Dr. Chopra do, in fact, conform to the **scientific evidence**. The best book I have seen on this subject is called *"The Balance Within - The Science Connecting Health and Emotions,"* by Esther M. Sternburg, M.D.

Published in 2000, this book states unequivocally that **stress does affect the immune system**. The medical "establishment" ridiculed this simple statement only a few years ago.

Dr. Sternburg describes her work as follows:

"The science of brain-immune system communications is by its very nature a field that does this [shows how one field of specialization can be applied to others to reweave the tapestry of the human body]. *It looks inward to the most detailed level of body chemistry and at the same time it looks outward to the larger concerns of health and emotion. It applies technologies that analyze molecules and genes with technologies that image the functioning of whole organs like the brain. It bridges specialized disciplines of basic science like immunology and neurobiology, and it bridges specialized fields of medicine such as psychiatry and rheumatology. It bridges the basic sciences with clinical medicine and both of these with the intangible but essential input of feeling and emotion. The end result is to make the body and mind whole again."*

Specifically, **immune system** molecules can and do cross the **"blood-brain barrier,"** previously thought to be impermeable, like the Great Wall of China. The result is that the **cytokines** (a particular kind of immune system molecule) do, in fact, **kill off neurons** in the brain and contribute to the slow loss of memory seen in dementia victims -- e. g. Alzheimer's disease, AIDS, senility, etc.

This means that **weakened immune systems** lead directly to **degenerative brain disorders**. Possibly quite soon, this knowledge will lead to **breakthroughs** in the treatment of these diseases.

On the other hand, this science is finding that **"believing can make you well."** Examples that **all physicians** have seen, such as "I'll fight this cancer one more month until my grandchild is born," have a scientific basis. The body's nerve and hormone responses to stimuli, which are controlled by the brain, do, in fact, **directly affect** our immune system.

Work can be a positive or negative experience. Conditioning can occur in either direction. If the environment is nurturing, supportive and rewarding, the **stress** associated with work becomes a **positive stimulus**. If the workplace is hostile and unsupportive, it can literally make us **sick from the stress**. Studies in a variety of disciplines prove this -- endocrinology, biochemistry, immunology, and psychology. Dr. Sternburg has documented them all in **very convincing fashion**. The bibliography at the end of her book documents hundreds of studies covering 14 pages.

We have all **experienced** this. It is **intuitive**. Any positive or negative emotion affects our immune system cells. Psychologists have proven again and again that **negative stress** leads directly to increased **vulnerability** to viral infections. **Grief**, for example, and the stress endured by caregivers of Alzheimer's and other terminal patients, correlate with **reduced** immune system function.

As Dr. Sternburg states, it was probably necessary to go through the period of **increasing specialization** from Descartes and Bacon until the **1960's** or so. Now, however, each scientific discipline is so **overwhelmed with detail** that focus on the parts has caused us to **lose sight of the whole**. In health, just now, the disciplines are beginning to come together to arrive at a

"unified theory," as sought in physics to explain the universe. We are not there yet, but this theory definitely includes an **interaction between the emotions and the immune system.**

Applying This Knowledge

So what, you say? What's in it for me? What should I do **differently**? Good questions, all.

There are at least **four major changes** you need to make in your life once you have acquired this knowledge:

> ➤ Change your **work environment**, if possible, to one that is **positive**. Easier said than done? Sure. But today there is infinitely more **flexibility** on when and where work gets done than **before the Internet**. Get **creative** about what you do and where you do it. Work at **home** as an **affiliate** to one or more web site promotions. **Telecommute**, if your work allows it. Change the **texture of your day** with breaks for workouts, meditation or just relaxing.

> ➤ If you are well, enhance your immune system with **positive interactions** with other people and the **joy of creation**. Join support groups. **Volunteer** at local hospice organizations or hospitals. Get started in **hobbies** that produce positive feedback -- painting, writing, golf, tennis, singing, etc.

> ➤ If you are **sick**, boost your **immune system** and take a healthy dose of vitamin, mineral and amino acid **supplements**. Eat a healthy diet low in carbohydrates or my version of the "Budwig diet" (Chapter 5).

> ➤ Build up to 30 to 60 minutes of **exercise** at least **4 days a week**. It is proven that regular exercise produces a flood

of positive feelings about yourself as well as building up your **stamina** and immune system. See the booklet on Exercise for some specific suggestions.

The Result

Once you have reached a **positive mental and physical state**, you'll know it. How? Well, here are some **measurements** for both your physical condition and your body that will help you tell when you're "there."

You will know that your body has reached its proper condition when:

➤ You can **walk two miles** in less than **twenty-four minutes**, and still maintain a conversation at the end of your walk.

➤ You **do not smoke**. You **limit your alcohol** to no more than one and a half ounces of whiskey or six ounces of wine per day.

➤ You **fall asleep readily** at night. You get an average of seven to seven and a half hours of sleep each night.

➤ Your weight falls within **5 percent** of your ideal body weight. These tables are available at any gym or health food store.

➤ Your **percent body fat** falls in the right range. If you are a man, your percent body fat is **8 to 12 percent**. If you are a woman, you have **15 to 18 percent** body fat. [Any gym can measure your body's fat percentage for you.]

You will know that your mental attitude is healthy when:

➢ You are doing exactly what you want to do in life and **feel generally happy**.

➢ You wake up each morning **feeling great**, not just good.

➢ You take **regular vacations**.

➢ You realize you are part of a large **mutual support system** and regularly **offer your support** to your family, friends and colleagues.

➢ You are committed to the basic **value of life** and see it as **worth living**.

➢ You believe you have a **mission in life** and that your mission fits into a purpose that connects with the family of man in a larger universe.

➢ You have a **sense of humor**. You can **laugh at yourself** when you find you take yourself too seriously.

Other clues that help you know you're healthy:

➢ You have **taken charge** of your health and health care. You realize that, like illness, excellent health is a **composite**, made up of many different components. You recognize that **you are responsible** for those components.

➢ You have worked to make your **immune system** an ally. It is finely tuned, ready and able to battle infectious agents of all types, seeking out and **destroying** abnormal cells that could lead to allergies, arthritis, diabetes or even **cancer**.

> You not only meet the **average stresses** of daily life **head-on**, you seek out challenges of your own. Even your **vacations** become physical **challenges**.

You have become an **informed consumer**. You carefully read the labels on all the food you eat and **understand** what those labels mean. You **co-doctor** intelligently, seeking knowledge on your own to help you **get and stay healthy.**

To Your Health!!

Booklet #2 – Stop Your Aging With Exercise

HEALTHY EXERCISE

What Ever Happened to Jim Fixx?

I'm sure there were lots of you who, as I did, wondered how a great runner and advocate of running for health purposes could **drop dead with a heart attack** as **Jim Fixx** did in 1984. Many of you are saying, "Who's Jim Fixx?"

I mention him only because he exemplifies the truism that **physical fitness** isn't everything. Jim Fixx was born in 1932, just like me. He published a book in 1977 called **"The Complete Book of Running."** He is credited with **starting** America's **fitness revolution**. Yet, he died in 1984 at age 52 practicing the sport he was an expert in. He had heart arteries **clogged with atherosclerosis**.

So what? Well, healthy exercise is **no guarantee** of either a long or a healthy life. So, can you couch potatoes **relax**? **No way!!**

Healthy exercise is an essential part of your **get and stay well lifestyle**. It is not just good for you. It is **essential**. However, it must be combined with **healthy eating habits**, which are also essential (see Booklet #1 above).

What is healthy exercise? That is the question I'm going to answer in this booklet. First, I **do not** recommend **running or jogging**. Why? It is hard to get someone to **gauge your progress**, particularly at first, and make sure you **don't overdo it**. Also, it is notoriously **hard on knees, ankles and feet** ... not just of us seniors, but of everyone.

A Step-by-Step Approach

STEP ONE: Get a membership in a gymnasium. Two reasons. Every good gym has people to **supervise** your initial attempts to **regain your fitness**. And second, once you begin paying for something like a gym membership, it's a **powerful incentive** to continue to use it. The typical price is $40 - 50 a month.

This is **not** your father's gym. In fact, the "politically correct" name for a gym nowadays is "health club" or "fitness center." I'll continue to use "gym", thank you.

If you haven't been in a gym for a while, go take a look. You will be pleasantly surprised. A good gym is **attractive, airy and air-conditioned.** You do not feel like it's just a sweatshop for muscle builders. The facilities are modern, quiet and **computerized**. There are TVs available to watch (with headsets for the audio) while you're doing your treadmill or bicycle aerobics. Some rent headsets to listen to the TV. Or, you can take your own earphone radio, as I do.

Most gym memberships involve a **contract** for some period of time. Typical is **two years.** These people aren't dummies. They know, as **Dr. Joe Davis** told me when I first joined his Ultra Fit gym, that once you exercise regularly for **three months**, you're **hooked**. You feel and look so good that you will continue it and **give it priority.**

Ideally, you join with a **friend or loved one**. You keep each other honest. But **don't** count on that. Your friend or loved one may not be as motivated as you are. Plan to **do it yourself**. Take your friend or loved one, if you can, but don't wait for that. We're talking about **your life** here.

 STEP TWO: Line up a **trainer** at the gym. If they don't have qualified trainers, look for a gym that does. Check this on the phone. Gyms are **competitive**, just like other businesses. Make them **prove the value** of their membership to you.

The gym may **provide you a trainer** for your first couple of workouts as part of the sign-up agreement. If not, the trainer will typically charge **$20 per hour**. You will need one for only the **first two weeks**. Plan on spending **$100** on the trainer.

During that time, the trainer will do an **assessment** of your fitness level, muscle **measurements** and fat percentage. They will outline a program for you to start a **comprehensive** exercise routine. They will check you out on how to use the weight-lifting machines -- another **prerequisite.** They will calculate for you a **maximum heart rate** to use as you begin using the **aerobic** machines. And, most important, they will **monitor** your first few workouts to make sure you are doing them **correctly**.

I will give you some **general guidelines** here. But there is **no substitute** for a trainer to get you familiar with all the **exercise options** to improve your fitness level. The trainer will show you how to **start slowly** enough so there is **no muscle pain**. No pain, no gain...**NOT!!** Your routine should include a mixture of **weight-bearing exercises** (circuit weights), **aerobics** (treadmill, bicycle, step climber, etc.) and **stretching**.

The gym should offer **periodic assessments** - fitness level, muscle measurements, fat percentage measurement and recommended exercises - **free**. Another **prerequisite**. Don't sign up without it.

STEP THREE: Join an aerobics class. This **jump-starts** the social aspect of going to the gym, which is **very important**. You need this to be a **pleasant experience.** You need the support of a group.

Any gym you join should have a **wide variety** of aerobics, Tae Kwan Do, jazzercise, yoga, etc. classes for you to choose from. One popular option involves using a large rubber ball to lie on in various positions to **stretch** your muscles. This absolutely needs to be done **with supervision** when you're starting.

STEP FOUR: **Just do it!!**

Can't I Do It At Home?

Sure you can. But **you won't**. Those fancy exercise machines you see on TV are useful only if you want **another "white elephant."** We have one in the storage closet. Take it from a **champion procrastinator**. Without the social and financial pressure of a **gym membership**, you will **not** exercise systematically and regularly.

In **1961**, the U. S. Air Force adopted a **British system of aerobic exercise** as its official fitness routine for all members. We were to do it **on our own, at home**. Did we do it? Sure. **Some of us. Some of the time**.

In **1967**, I heard a lecture at Randolph Air Force Base in San Antonio by **Dr. Kenneth Cooper**. At that time, he was a Captain in the Air Force. He has since become **famous** for his fitness clinic in Dallas, where he works with seriously ill people, particularly those with **heart problems**.

The Air Force adopted Dr. Cooper's program as its **official exercise routine** for all members. We were to do it **on our own, at home**. Did we do it? Sure. **Some of us. Some of the time.**

Believe me, this is one rut that I've fallen in enough times that you can **use my experience to avoid it**. Isn't that what we all hope **our kids** will do? Do they do it? **Some of them. Some of the time....**

Well, you get the idea. Get started on a **supervised routine** of exercise **now**. Whatever **age** you are. However much **money** or time you have or don't have. It's the only way that works long-term.

What Specifically Does a Good Workout Routine Look Like?

Let me describe mine for you. I do this 3 or 4 times a week. Remember, I built up to this level over a period of about **two years**. At first, I did a **very modest** version of this. I was **60** at the time, in 1992.

My experience before this with regular gym workouts was limited to my Air Force days and **a few months** when I was in my mid-50s. At that time, I did not have any **social support** and the gym environment **wasn't friendly** and I quit.

My workout takes **about an hour** and breaks down into **four parts**:

1. Warm-up. I ride the stationary bike for five minutes. It has various levels of pedal resistance. I use one that gets my pulse up to about 120 beats per minute and loosens up my muscles.

2. Circuit Weights. These are **computerized** weight machines -- 12 of them. When I come in, I punch in my **member number** at the central computer. Then, when I get to each machine, I punch the number in again and it **"remembers"** how much weight I used in my **last workout**.

This is the major advantage of computerized circuit weight machines. You don't have to **remember** where you were last time. It also **automatically** adds a certain percentage (varies by machine) to your weight for the negative (back to GO) stroke. The first three and last three repetitions are at a lower weight, to get you started and ease you back to normal at the end (nice, but not essential).

Also, at anytime, you can get **a printout** of your history of workouts -- first workout, best workout, most recent workout, etc. with the **weights for each**. I do **2 sets** of **12 repetitions each** on each of the 12 circuit weight machines. Here is my latest workout:

> Leg Press 132 lbs positive/152 lbs negative
> Leg Curl 84 lbs positive/117 lbs negative
> Leg Extension 70 lbs positive/98 lbs negative
> Chest Press 119 lbs positive/166 negative
> Lat Pulldown 82 lbs positive/103 lbs negative
> Fly 69 lbs positive/86 lbs negative
> Seated Row 109 lbs positive/152 lbs negative
> Shoulder Press 50 lbs positive/63 lbs negative
> Arm Curl 30 lbs positive/42 lbs negative
> Tricep Extension 37 lbs positive/46 lbs negative
> Abdominal 96 lbs positive/120 lbs negative
> Back Extension 130 lbs positive/163 lbs negative

Does that make you tired just looking at it? **You can do it, too**. I have added some muscle mass, but not a lot. Obviously, ladies, you would need **less weight** to maintain your muscle strength...but you, too, **need** this. It's not just a guy thing.

Mostly what this does is build up your **muscle tone**, and strengthen your tendons, ligaments and everything else that will help keep you **free** of joint problems, arthritis, diabetes (see Booklet #3 on diabetes) and all sorts of other degenerative disease problems.

3. Abdominal/Back Exercises. Next, I do a group of exercises designed to strengthen my **abdominal** and **lower back muscles**. These have cured a **chronic back pain** I suffered from in my 50s. By 1992 when I started regularly exercising, the pain included **extreme shooting pain** down my right sciatic nerve. The sciatic nerve runs from your hip area down the back of each leg.

There are **five types** of exercise. Each helps in a different way. I have had only occasional **mild twinges** in my lower back since 1992. These usually occur after I have **missed a week or so** at the gym due to a heavy slate of commitments. I now do these exercises **almost every day**, wherever I am. They can be done on the carpeted floor anywhere **in the house or a hotel room**. They require no equipment. Try them; you'll like them!

> **Partial Sit-ups ("crunches").** Lie on the floor (mat) on your back with your feet flat on the floor (knees raised). With your hands on opposite shoulders (right on left, left on right), raise your head and shoulders a few inches off the mat. Return to the start position. I do 30 - 35 of these. You should start with **no more than 10**. Increase at the rate of **5 more per week**. In time, you can begin lifting your shoulders higher off the mat, but **never to a full sit-up position**.

Oblique Sit-ups. The oblique muscles are very important in toning up your abdominal muscles (which **erase back pain**). They run vertically down the outside of your abdomen, on both sides.

First, from the same start position as for the Partial Sit-ups above, place your right ankle on your left knee. Place your left hand behind your head. Keep your right hand flat on the mat. Raise your **left elbow** to touch your **right knee**. Again, start with 10 repetitions. Reverse positions and raise your **right elbow** to touch your **left knee.** Add no more than 5 repetitions per week. As you gain muscle tone, you can make the exercise a little harder by placing your calf and finally your knee on the other knee instead of your ankle. I do 30-35 of these with my knee on my other knee.

Leg Lifts. From the same start position as the Sit-ups, **raise your legs** (with knees bent) toward your chest. At the highest position, be sure your **butt is off the mat** and your feet are together. Slowly **lower your legs** until they are **10 inches or so** off the mat and then **raise them again**. Do only 3 or 4 of these to start. Add one per week. I do 20 of these.

Legs to Chest. Finally, an exercise that a Physical Therapist showed me 18 years ago. She said that if I did **25 of these every day**, I would **never again** have back problems. **She was right**.

Begin in the same position as for the Sit-ups. Raise **both legs together** (with knees bent) until they are as **close to your chest** as possible. Grasp them with both arms and hold for a **six second count**. Lower them to the floor and repeat the exercise. Do **no more than 8** of these to begin. Add 1 or 2 per week. I do 35 of these.

When you get up from the mat, **be cautious**. It is common to **be dizzy** at first as your circulation readjusts to the vertical position. Sit down with your **head between your knees** for a couple of minutes until the dizziness goes away.

4. Aerobic Exercise. So far, except for the warm-up, the exercises have been designed to **strengthen and-or stretch** your muscles. Essential to your fitness routine is a session of **aerobic** exercise. Most experts say that for optimum gain, you need to **elevate your heart rate to 80 percent** of your maximum and keep it there for **at least 20 minutes**. Do this at least 3 times a week.

What is your maximum heart rate? You and your **trainer** will figure that out at the **first session.** There is a standardized table based on your age. But, like the standardized weight tables, there is a **lot of variation** based on blood pressure, heart condition, level of fitness and **other variables**. Don't try this at home!!

For the aerobic part of my workout, which if you **insist** on ranking them, is **probably the most important**, I use the treadmill. It is the most popular of the aerobic machines at the gym I go to. Probably, that is because of the **wide variation** of routines available (and the convenience of their location in front of the bank of TV screens).

I use a **heart rate option** on the computerized machines at my gym. That means you can **set the maximum heart rate** you and your trainer have figured out. You also enter your body weight, the speed you want and the number of minutes for your workout. The machine then **figures out the elevation** of the treadmill necessary to produce that heart rate for you.

It **continually monitors** your heart rate through a set of handles that you grasp during the workout. When your heart rate has reached your desired maximum, the machine **automatically** adjusts the elevation to keep it there. If it has lowered it to level (zero degrees of elevation) and your actual heart rate is **too high**, it will tell you to **reduce your speed** (from 4.0 to 3.5 miles per hour, for example) so the maximum heart rate can be maintained.

Also included on the treadmill (and the bicycle and stair climber) is a **"fitness test."** This will put you through a five minute drill using varying elevations and give you a **readout** on how you did (poor, average, good or excellent) based on your heart rate.

At the end of your workout, the machine will go through a one-minute "cool down" period at reduced speed and elevation designed to **gradually** get your heart rate back to normal.

I do **22 minutes 3 or 4 times a week** with the maximum heart rate set at **125 beats per minute**. That is the "standard" maximum for a person 47 years old. One of the trainers recommended that level after a fitness test.

Summary

The routine I have described above takes me **almost exactly one hour**. I try to do it in the morning, but you can do it **anytime**. Most modern gyms are open 24/7. The level I've reached **required about two years** of gradual buildup. Since then (1994), I have remained at a **"maintenance"** level of fitness.

You can certainly do as well or better than I did. **Challenge yourself**. But, above all, don't **get in a hurry** to reach some particular level of fitness. This is a **lifelong highway.** There will be signposts along the way, but you will continue traveling down it **as long as you live**.

Because of it, you will live longer. Dr. Roizen's book, *Real Age*, estimates that my level of exercise adds three years to my life or reduces my "Real Age", in his terms, by three years. More important than that, **I feel great**.

I play **golf twice a week,** weather permitting. I have **no muscle or joint pain**.

I feel full of energy and stamina every morning. At least once, sometimes twice, a week I stand on the "risers" and **sing with a men's chorus for 2 1/2 to 3 hours**. I play bridge on the computer with people from all over the world.

I enjoy **vacations** with my family about three times a year, plus weekend excursions. I am happier than ever before in my life (thanks largely to Terry, my beautiful wife) and I feel much **younger than I did 40 years ago.**

GENERAL GUIDELINES ABOUT EXERCISE

Here are several general guidelines for you to keep in mind when you exercise. Your **trainer** may give you more.

1. **Breathe out** during the **positive** stroke of each exercise. That is, take a breath just before you start. For the weight machines, it is **obvious** what the positive stroke is. It's the **first thing you do** during each repetition, whether it's the Fly, the Seated Row or whatever. **Do not hold your breath.** This will avoid a hernia in a muscle in your abdomen. Breathing in will occur normally on the negative

stroke. To **avoid hyperventilation**, purse your lips as you breathe out. This will slow it down.

On the floor exercises (partial sit-ups, etc.), the positive stroke is also the first thing you do during each repetition. As you lift your head and shoulders, for example, you should be **breathing out**.

During the aerobics portion of your routine, it is a good idea to adopt a **rhythmic breathing pattern**. For example, breathe in for four steps on the treadmill, and breathe out for six steps. This will help build up the **oxygen carrying capacity** of your lungs.

2. Perform the exercises **slowly**. **Don't** try to show off as the "Macho Man/Superwoman" and do each repetition as fast as you can. You get **much more effect** from the same number of repetitions if you do them slowly.

3. **Accent the Negative**. Experts say the negative stroke in each exercise contributes 80% of the value of that exercise. This is not intuitive. This is why the computerized weight machines add a **percentage more weight** during the negative stroke. In addition, you should consciously take longer to do this negative stroke than the positive stroke. If you do the **positive** in a **count of two**, do the **negative** in a **count of four**.

4. Increase the weight until you feel you can **just barely complete** the last repetition on that machine. Exception: **if you feel pain, stop!** It's quite simple to increase the weight on the computerized circuit weight machines. The idea is to **continue stressing** your muscles as they develop strength and stamina.

For the floor exercises, the same principle applies. At the end of each set, you should feel like you could not possibly do another repetition.

5. Keep your muscles **stressed** all the time during your exercises. In other words, **don't relax between repetitions**. The idea is to tone up your muscles as quickly as possible **without pain**. That occurs when you **maintain the stress** on your muscle between repetitions.

6. If you miss **a week or so** (because of illness or whatever), assume that your progress has been set back **three weeks**. When you start again, try to go back to where you were **three weeks before**. If you miss three weeks or more, assume you are starting over from scratch.

NOTE: As you pursue the routines of diet and exercise in this book, you will be pleasantly surprised that the colds, flu and other common maladies you have been used to **quietly disappear** from your life.

7. Anytime you feel pain of any kind, **STOP**. No well-planned and executed exercise routine should be painful. The pain is warning you that you are **overdoing** whatever you are doing. Stop. Take a rest and try it again at a lower stress/weight level. If the pain persists, **bypass** that exercise completely for a few days until you can perform it without pain.

NOTE: It is a good idea to **weigh yourself** every time you go to the gym. Just remember, **muscle weighs more** than fat. If you are not losing weight as fast as you like, it could be because your muscles are **"bulking up."** This is also a great excuse when you don't lose a pound or so a week!

Also, don't forget to measure your waist (at the largest point) periodically. Several doctors have told me that the best indicator of what they call **"Metabolic Syndrome"** (a collection of symptoms which lead to diabetes and other maladies) is **waist size**. For females, the maximum is **35 inches**; for males, it is **40 inches**. Don't cheat. Measure the largest circumference.

Best of luck, and remember...**Just do it!**

Booklet #3 – Beating Diabetes

DIABETES

Do you **know someone** who suffers from **diabetes**? Do **you** suffer from it? For most of us, it's **one or the other**.

A recent article by Erin McClam, distributed by Associated Press and published in the San Antonio Express-News pointed out that diabetes increased at an **alarming rate** in the United States during the **past decade**. It has risen **70 percent** among people **in their 30s**. Nationally, the share of the population diagnosed with diabetes jumped **33 percent** between 1990 and 1998.

What's even more frightening is that a recent study published by the UK Prospective Diabetes Study suggests that before most patients are actually diagnosed with Type II diabetes (also called "adult-onset diabetes"), the pancreas has lost its ability to properly control post-meal blood sugar levels **for over 8 years** and insulin resistance has been present for **up to 12 years**.

Until recently, the earliest Type II diabetes was seen in those in their 40s or older. That has changed **dramatically**. In the last few years, an alarming number of children have been diagnosed with Type II diabetes. Type II is appearing more frequently in pre-pubescent children, and has even been documented in children as young as **four years old** (American Diabetes Foundation).

The cause? Very simple. **Obesity**. The nation's weight problem is well documented. The number of Americans considered obese **soared** from about one in eight in 1991 to over **one in four** today.

Some **20 million** Americans have diabetes, and the number is expected to rise to **22 million** by 2025. And remember, this is counting only those who have been **diagnosed** with diabetes...not the millions who have it but are **unaware** of it.

According to the American Diabetic Association, almost **25 percent** of Mexican-Americans between the ages of 45 and 74 have diabetes. In San Antonio, where I used to live, local health officials say **120,000 residents** either had diabetes or were at risk of developing the disease. In 35 years of personal observation of San Antonians, it was increasingly **hard for me to find** an adult Mexican-American (62% of our population in San Antonio) who was **not obese**.

The Cause -- Details

Let's take a **more detailed look** at why you or your loved one has diabetes. I cannot improve on the explanation published by Dr. David Williams (remember him?) in his newsletter *Alternatives* in August 2000. This newsletter with a **long article** titled *"Sugar is Slow Suicide"* is available at his web site: http://www.DrDavidWilliams.com

*"For decades 'health nuts,' including yours truly, have been warning about the **dangers** of increased **sugars** and/or **refined carbohydrates** in the diet.*

*Let me tell you, it has been a **real uphill battle** trying to convince the public that consuming **too much sugar** could eventually lead to diabetes -- especially when **conventional** medicine kept*

asserting that sugar is **totally harmless**. Even today, as diabetes reaches epidemic proportions in this country, most doctors continue to preach that dietary sugar has **no connection** to behavior problems, mood swings, depression, or the **increased incidence of adult onset diabetes**.

Our **FDA** says that the **only problem** sugar causes is **dental caries**. And with the support of the American Dietetic Association, the **Sugar Association** has stuck to the position that at only 15 calories per teaspoon, sugar is a **healthy, low-calorie sweetener** that is no different than any other carbohydrate. Nothing could be **further from the truth**. In fact, **decades of research** support the fact that a 'sweet tooth' will **invariably** lead to a lifetime of poor health and a **premature death**.

The carbohydrates we eat are converted by the body into a simple sugar called **glucose**. This glucose, or 'blood sugar,' enters the **blood stream** to be transported throughout the body. **Blood sugar** is the **primary energy source** used by the brain, the nervous system, and the muscles. To be utilized, the blood sugar must get from the bloodstream **into the nerve and muscle cells**. This is where **insulin** comes into the picture. As I'm sure many of you recall from high school biology, insulin is the **pancreatic hormone** that opens up the cell walls so blood sugar can enter. It is the **key** to the whole energy process. Insulin is **secreted** in **two phases**. A surge of insulin is initially released **immediately following a meal**, or when sugar or sweetness is detected in the mouth and digestive system. A **second round** of insulin is released shortly after a meal and **continues to be released gradually** for several hours.

For insulin to work properly, it must be present in **sufficient quantities**, and the **cells** in your body must be **'sensitive'** to its effects. When cells don't react to the effects of insulin by allowing *sugar to enter through their cell walls, a condition called __insulin resistance__ exists. Insulin resistance **isn't fully understood** at this point. However, we **do know** that __insulin resistance is often directly related to obesity.__ This is especially true when a person has a fat build-up in the **waist or abdominal area.***

*Studies have shown that obese, non-diabetic individuals can reduce their levels of circulating insulin **simply by losing weight**. This reduction in the amount of insulin occurs **without any changes** in blood sugar levels. In other words, by **losing weight**, one can often **overcome** insulin resistance. This is true because, with **less fat** to complicate the picture, existing insulin levels become **more effective** at lowering blood sugar levels.*

*On the flip side of this coin, excess abdominal fat and fat that has been accumulated **around the liver** increase the amount of circulating free fatty acids in the blood. As these fatty acids break down, they **increase toxicity levels**. In turn, increased toxicity has been shown to do two things: First, it **inhibits** the **production** of insulin; and second, it makes muscle cells **less sensitive** to the insulin that is available. Muscle tissue is **crucial** in helping to balance blood sugar levels. Under normal circumstances, over **80 percent** of the blood sugar released immediately following a meal is taken up by **muscle cells**.*

A Wrench in the Works

*It should be obvious from this simple biology review that the **regulation of insulin** is a **very** important part of staying healthy and alive. Unfortunately, an **increasing percentage** of the American population cannot maintain this balance. And when their insulin and blood sugar regulation capabilities get **seriously out of whack**, their condition is referred to as **diabetes**."*

Well, so much for the cause of this insidious, silent killer. Let's take a look at how you treat it once you or your loved one have been diagnosed with it.

Treating Diabetes

Dr. Williams gives us some **priceless** advice about what to do about it.

*"Most doctors fail to tell their patients that, even if they use the **best** conventional therapies available, type II diabetes will only get **progressively worse**. If your doctor has led you to believe that taking your prescription medication will either **fix your diabetes** or keep it from getting worse, you've been **terribly misinformed**. When you look at the current treatment programs, this shouldn't come as any surprise.*

*The whole idea in treating diabetes is to bring fluctuating blood sugar levels back to normal **as quickly as possible**. This must be done immediately after eating and then **gradually continue** for several hours, as food is being digested. In non-diabetic individuals, this process occurs **very smoothly** because the body constantly **adjusts** its secretion of insulin depending on the levels of blood sugar....*

*...Using either of these **drug** types [stimulating insulin production; and various newer drug types] is a **shotgun approach** at best. When **too little insulin** is released, blood sugar levels rise, causing the formation of **triglycerides and fat storage**. When there's **too much insulin**, blood sugar levels begin to fall (hypoglycemia), triggering a **feeling of hunger** and the constant need to eat, which also **causes weight gain and fat storage.***

*...These problems explain why diabetics treated with **oral medications** ... have a **weight gain** of anywhere from **6 to 12 pounds or more**. And, as I explained earlier, this weight gain and the extra deposits of fat become part of the vicious cycle that causes diabetes to **progressively worsen.***

*Additionally, the **roller-coaster effect** from constantly fluctuating blood sugar levels contributes to increased blood fats, high blood pressure, increased stickiness of the blood and clot formation, heart failure, poly-cystic ovary disease, nerve pain and degeneration, and damage to the small blood vessels, especially those in the eyes, the kidneys, and the lower limbs.*

*Before you place **complete trust** in your medication to take care of your diabetes problem, take a look at this list of **complications** linked directly to progressing diabetes. It comes from the **American Diabetes Foundation**.*

Diabetes is now:

- ➤ *the **leading cause of blindness** in people age 20 to 74*
- ➤ *the **leading cause of kidney failure***
- ➤ *the **leading cause of amputation of the lower limbs***
- ➤ *responsible for 50 to 60 percent of the **impotence** problems in males over the age of 50*
- ➤ *responsible for **severe nerve damage** in 60 to 70 percent of all diabetics*
- ➤ *the **major cause of stroke** in the United States*
- ➤ *known to increase the **risk of heart disease** by 2 to 4 times over normal. (In the UKPDS study I mentioned earlier, researchers found that even when intensive efforts were made to control blood sugar levels in diabetics, the risk of developing heart problems was not affected. **Diabetics without any previous history of heart attack had the***

same high heart attack risk as non-diabetics with a previous heart attack.)

Diabetes is one of those diseases that can make the treating doctor look **like an absolute genius.** After placing a patient on diabetic medication, the doctor can predict with **uncanny accuracy** the chain of health problems that will begin to develop **like clockwork** in the upcoming years. Keep in mind, the chain of events will happen **even if you comply** perfectly with the therapy. In essence, the doctors can predict the **progressive decline** -- but do nothing to prevent it.

An Epidemic in the Making

The increasing incidence of diabetes creates a **perfect marketing target** for pharmaceutical companies. Just look at the facts -- and the trends.

Diabetes is a **growing epidemic** in this country, with **no end in sight.** Adult-onset diabetes has increased between **600 percent** and **1,000 percent** in the last 60 years. It is currently increasing at a rate of **6 percent a year,** and that rate is **expected to accelerate.**

Currently, **one in every five** American kids is obese. And since obesity is directly linked to diabetes, the **target population** for diabetic pharmaceuticals now extends clear down to **four-year olds.** Yes, diabetes is a pharmaceutical company's **dream come true.**

As I said before, pharmaceutical companies are the **best marketers** in the world -- but don't get caught up in believing that they have the magic bullet for diabetes. That would be a **fatal mistake.** Diabetes is a disease in which you have to address several **underlying factors.**

Muscle Up to Help Control Blood Sugar

*First and foremost, the most important factor is to get your weight down. In **almost every case** of type II diabetes, the body can control blood sugar fluctuations **naturally** when the **obesity problem** is taken care of. Obviously, this will require both **changes in the diet** and at least **moderate amounts of exercise**.*

Exercise provides you with four important benefits. It
➢ *increases lean body tissue*
➢ *burns fat*
➢ *increases the sensitivity of insulin, enabling the pancreas to produce less,*
➢ *and raises the metabolic rate."*

Artificial Sweeteners

One final comment before we leave the subject of diabetes. Don't be fooled into thinking that the use of **Sweet and Low, Equal**, etc. sweeteners "help" control your blood sugar. If you are a diabetic, the only artificial sweeteners you should use are **stevia, agave nectar or xylitol.** They are now **widely available** in health food stores. Here's an e-mail from the wife of a diabetic to Dr. Williams:

*"My husband is diabetic. He drinks 4 or 5 cups of blueberry tea every day. We sweeten it with **stevia.** It keeps his sugar controlled. He started taking the tea steadily about a year ago, and gradually the doctor saw the **good numbers** that my husband recorded for his **sugar reading** each day. His medicine was **decreased by half**, then a few months later, **all**. Stevia*

does not have the same effect on the pancreas as does sugar, Sweet and Low, or Equal.

Dorothy D."

From The Local Newspaper

Remember my describing the high rates of diabetes among the Mexican-American population in San Antonio? Following is an article from the *San Antonio Express-News* by Paul Elizondo, County Commissioner for Precinct 2 in Bexar County (the county that includes San Antonio). He titled it ***"Do yourself a favor: Get a diabetes test."***

"I scheduled a doctor's appointment because I had this terrible rash that was really ugly. After the doctor ran a blood test, he came in and said, 'Congratulations, you have diabetes. At last, you'll have to do what I tell you or there will be consequences!'

That was about four years ago, and the disease has taken its toll on me, particularly on my eyesight.

*I have Type 2 diabetes; years ago, it was called adult onset diabetes. In many instances, it can be controlled with the proper diet and exercise, but **my busy schedule makes it difficult.***

I know there are thousands of San Antonians like me who have demanding jobs. My days run long into the night, like when we were working on the contract for the new arena, which required 16- to 18-hour days.

*Plus, I have my own band, meaning I work two jobs. I try to walk three miles every other day and eat planned meals, but many days **I just can't do it**.*

These are some of the excuses we conjure up for not changing our lifestyles. But when we look at the potential consequences of diabetes – blindness, stroke, heart and kidney failure and limb amputation – it's a no-brainer: Change lifestyle or perish!

The first step is awareness. San Antonio has a diabetes epidemic and I urge everybody to take advantage of free screenings today and Saturday.

The screenings are hosted by the Diabetes Alliance of Bexar County. The collaborative is hoping to screen 25,000 people all around town this week. In this city, there are approximately 80,000 people who have diabetes – and they don't even know it!

The alliance includes the Texas Diabetes Institute, American Diabetes Association and the Juvenile Diabetes Foundation and is dedicated to awareness, education, prevention and treatment of diabetes.

By marshalling their forces and convincing residents to take control of their health, perhaps we can help stem the tide of this deadly disease.

My best advice is to look at the risk factors. Do you have family members with diabetes? Are you Hispanic, Native American, Asian or African-American? Are you overweight? Do you have a bad diet? Do you love sweets and drink too many sodas? Do you drink too much and exercise too little?

Then, my friend, you are a prime candidate for diabetes.

If you love your family and if you love yourself, you need to be screened as soon as possible. There is nothing more insidious to our families than diabetes.

Look at the odds. Are you among the 80,000 walking around who don't know they have diabetes? Get screened today. Call xxx-xxxx for times and locations."

Commissioner Elizondo has given you good advice. Remember, it is never too late to begin treating your diabetes with proper diet and exercise. Your miracle immune system will restore your God-given body to normal functioning, if you'll just give it the support it needs.

God Bless You!!

Booklet #4 – Cure Your Back Pain

BACK PROBLEMS

TMS -- An Interesting Mind-Body Connection

Back pain and, to a lesser extent, shoulder and neck pain, are common complaints. Around **80%** of the U.S. population has some history of one or the other. It is the first cause of **worker absenteeism** in this country. It ranks second behind respiratory infections as a reason for a **doctor visit**. An article in Forbes magazine in August 1986 reported that **$56 billion** are spent annually to deal with the consequences of back and neck pain. It's **much higher now**, you can be sure.

Doctors **cannot** see pain. Thus, theories about what **causes** back and neck pain are just that - **theories**. At best, an operation to "fix" a **"slipped disc"** in your spine is a **guess** that it is causing your pain. There is a great deal of evidence that many of the **operations** done on the spine **are unnecessary**.

Back in **1985,** Dr. Hubert Rosomoff, a well known neurosurgeon and chairman of his department at the University of Miami School of Medicine, published an article titled *"Do Herniated Discs Produce Pain?"* Dr. Rosomoff did **back operations** for many years. His conclusions were **based on logic** as well as his experience. He said that **continued compression** on a nerve would cause it to **stop** transmitting pain messages after a **short time**. The result is **numbness**. How could the herniated disc then cause **continuing pain**? His answer. **It couldn't**.

Chiropractors do **"adjustments"** on your back. They can't see pain, either. In most cases, in my experience, back pain sufferers who go to chiropractors achieve only **temporary relief**. The same can be said for massage therapists, Reiki practitioners, Rolfing, Voodoo and....well, **you name it**.

For me, **exercise** has been the "magic bullet" which **permanently** cured my back pain. Possibly, the **reduced stress** of my present life style **contributed** to the "cure." I don't know.

My former wife, Marge, had **chronic muscle spasms** in her shoulders and neck that caused **almost unbearable pain**. No doctor was able to fix it. A physical therapist gave her some **relief**, but only **temporary**. She was under **constant stress** over the shenanigans of her irresponsible daughter and grandchildren.

My experience tells me that the following study of the **cause and cure** for back pain (and neck and shoulder pain) is pretty close to the **real truth**. "Tension Myositis Syndrome (TMS)" is the name given to most of these pains by John E. Sarno, M.D. in his book "*Healing Back Pain -- The Mind-Body Connection.*" Published in 1991, this book **preceded** most of the research on the interaction of the mind and body documented by **Dr. Sternberg** and covered in Booklet #1 on Diet. The first edition of Dr. Sarno's book in 1984 also preceded **Dr. Chopra's** inspired insights about the **mind-body connection**.

What Causes Back and Neck Pain?

Dr. Sarno says the cause is **repressed emotions**. Further, that the pain acts as **camouflage** so that you and I don't have to deal with the **psychological pain** of making these repressed emotions conscious. I can't just dismiss this theory, and I hope you don't either. It is the result of **26 years** of treatment of

thousands of patients suffering from back and neck pain. Dr. Sarno's experience began as **director** of outpatient services at the Howard A. Rusk **Institute of Rehabilitation Medicine** at New York University Medical Center. He says:

*"**Conventional** medical training had taught me that these pains were primarily due to a variety of **structural abnormalities** of the spine, most commonly arthritic and disc disorders, or to a vague group of **muscle conditions** attributed to poor posture, underexercise, overexertion and the like.*

*...The experience of treating these patients was **frustrating** and depressing; one could **never** predict the outcome. Further, it was troubling to realize that the **pattern** of pain and physical examination findings often **did not correlate** with the presumed reason for the pain. For example, pain might be attributed to degenerative arthritic changes at the lower end of the spine but the patient might have pain in places that had **nothing to do** with the bones in that area. Or someone might have a lumbar disc that was herniated to the left and have pain in the right leg.*

*Along with the **doubt** about the accuracy of conventional diagnoses there came the realization that the **primary tissue** involved was muscle, specifically the muscles of the neck, shoulders, back and buttocks. But even more important was the observation that **88 percent** of the people seen had histories of such things as tension or migraine headache, heartburn, hiatus hernia, stomach ulcer, colitis, spastic colon, irritable bowel syndrome, hay fever, asthma, eczema and a variety of other disorders, all of which were **strongly suspected** of being related to **tension**. It seemed logical to conclude that their painful muscle condition might **also** be induced by tension. Hence the Tension Myositis Syndrome (TMS). (Myo means 'muscle;' Tension Myositis Syndrome is defined here as a change of state in the muscle that is painful.)*

*What do doctors think of this diagnosis? It is **unlikely** that most physicians are **aware of it**. I have written a number of medical papers and chapters for textbooks on the subject but they have **reached a limited medical audience**, primarily physicians working in the field of physical medicine and rehabilitation. In recent years it has become **impossible** to have medical papers on TMS accepted for publication, undoubtedly because these concepts **fly in the face** of **contemporary medical dogma**. For those physicians who might see this book, I would point out that it is **more complete** than any of the papers I have published and will be useful to them despite the fact it is written for a general audience.*

*The primary purpose of this book is to **raise the consciousness** both inside and outside the field of medicine, because these common pain syndromes represent a **major public health problem** that will not be solved until there is a change in the **medical perception** of their cause.*

*Having stated the purpose of the book, I would be less than candid if I did not report that many readers of its predecessor, Mind Over Back Pain, reported amelioration or **complete resolution** of symptoms. This substantiates the idea that it is **identification with** and **knowledge of** the disorder which are the **critical** therapeutic factors.*

[Here is just one example of Dr. Sarno's many patients.]

*The patient was a middle-aged woman with a grown-up family; she had been essentially **bedridden** for about **two years** when she came to my attention. She had suffered from low back and leg pain **for years**, had been **operated on twice**, and had gradually deteriorated to the point where her life was **restricted** almost entirely to her upstairs bedroom.*

*She was admitted to the hospital where we found **no evidence** of a continuing structural problem but **severe manifestations of TMS**. And no wonder, for the psychological evaluation revealed that she had endured terrible **sexual and psychological abuse** as a child and that she was in a **rage**, to put it mildly, and had **no awareness of it**. She was a pleasant, motherly sort of woman, the kind that would automatically **repress anger**. And so it **festered** in her for years, always **kept in check** by the severe pain syndrome.*

*Her recovery was stormy, for as the details of her life came out and she began to acknowledge her **fury**, she experienced a **variety of physical symptoms** -- cardiocirculatory, gastrointestinal, allergic -- but the pain **began to recede**. Group and individual psychotherapy was intense. Fortunately, she was **very intelligent** and grasped the concepts of TMS quickly. As the pain reduced, the staff helped to get her mobile again. Fourteen weeks after admission she went home essentially **free of pain** and ready to resume her life again."*

It's NOT All In Your Mind

Dr. Sarno is **not** saying, "It's all in your mind." Far from it. He points out that pain can be a **strong warning sign** of real **physical problems**. Your doctor should rule all these out before you begin to suspect that it is TMS.

In the last chapter of his book, Dr. Sarno reprints 10 long letters from his patients. They are **emotionally charged** and very convincing. I do not have room here to quote all 10. I've selected **one** that is quite **typical**. Remember, Dr. Sarno was doing this work in the **early 1980's**. None of the **scientific data** that today is confirming the mind-body **physical connection** was available. Here's the letter:

"Dear Dr. Sarno:

I want to thank you for how much you have helped my health and therefore the quality of my life....

*I had been suffering from severe back pain (both upper and lower, including sciatic) for **seven years** at the time I called you. I also had regular severe intestinal cramps, intense sharp pains in my chest; pain in my knees, ankles, elbows, wrists, knuckles and one shoulder.*

*All this pain, especially the back pain, **severely limited** my ability to work and play. I could not sweep the floor, do dishes, pick up babies (or anything over about three pounds, for that matter), join in sports, etc. Even brushing my hair hurt.*

*I had been a very strong, active person with a great need to exert myself physically -- which I (and everyone else) **blamed** as the **cause** of my back problems.*

*On the first visit to my doctor, I was told to **back off** as much activity as possible, to **do nothing** that hurt, and that probably a lot of things would hurt.*

*I followed that advice. Over the next seven years, I became an 'expert' on the supposed causes and cures of back pain, but **to no avail**. I had fourteen sessions of acupuncture, seventeen chiropractic sessions, seventeen 'body balancing' sessions, thirteen rolfing sessions, several physical therapy sessions, used a 'neuro-block TENS unit,' attended 'bad-back exercise class,' joined a health spa -- went swimming and used a Jacuzzi and sauna, received many massages, etc. One doctor thought it might be 'primary fibromyalgia syndrome' and tried putting me on L-Tryptophan and B6.*

All these treatments seemed to help a little at the time, but I still continued to suffer incredible pain.

*After my conversation with you, I considered seeing a psychotherapist, but I decided to try it without one first. I came to realize that it was not one big underlying problem causing my tension, but instead **any little thing** in my daily life that I had **learned to fear and/or that caused tension**, would begin my cycle of pain, more tension, more pain, etc. If the cause was an unresolved psychological conflict, I noticed that most of the time I didn't actually have to **resolve it** for the pain to go away but instead just be <u>**aware**</u> that this was the source of my pain. But I do find that now I tend to resolve things more quickly than I did before.*

*I was so mind-blown and happy over the ability to turn a **wrenching spasm** into a signal that something must be bothering me (emotionally or mentally) and then **dissolve the pain** completely within a matter of a minute or less.*

*It took me four months to get the process under good control, and within **less than a year,** I was able to say to friends and family, 'Yes, my back is finally **cured.** I am free of pain!'*

*At the same time that my back became free of pain, so did **every single other body part** that I mentioned earlier. Finally I could work and play again like I had not done for seven years. **What a relief!***

*I will always be grateful to you, Dr. Sarno, for having the courage and kindness to do what you've been doing for over **twenty years** -- helping people become **permanently** free of disabling pain.*

Thank you."

Ancient History

Most of us reading the above for the first time will consider this a new idea. **Wrong!** Dr. Sarno points out that **Hippocrates** himself, **2,500 years ago**, advised his **asthmatic patients** to be wary of **anger.**

*"In the late nineteenth century the famous French neurologist Jean-Martin Charcot gave new life to the principle of the interacting mind and body when he shared with the medical world his experiences with a group of intriguing patients. Called hysterics, they had dramatic neurological symptoms, like paralysis of an arm or leg, with **no evidence of neurological disease**. Imagine the effect on his medical audience, however, when he demonstrated that the paralysis could be **made to disappear** when the patient was **hypnotized!** One could not ask for a more convincing demonstration of the mind-body connection."*

Dr. Sarno describes the current medical "establishment" as under the thrall of **Rene Descartes (1596-1650).** Descartes' theories about the **separateness** of mind and body still drive most medical thought **today.** The body is the **purview of physicians** and all their technology. The mind is the **purview of psychologists and psychiatrists.** A significant number of doctors in the U. S. and most of them in Europe and other countries have **grown beyond** this view since 1991, when Dr. Sarno wrote it.

This mindset still persists in many doctors. It has led to reliance on **chemical "cures"** for mind and body illness. This, of course, **delights** the pharmaceutical companies. Many doctors still **treat symptoms** rather than **seeking out the causes**.

As for **"mind-body interaction,"** most doctors even today consider it folklore or **voodoo.**

Confirmation is Here

As far as acceptance by the medical "establishment", **little has changed** in the years since Dr. Sarno's observation above. You and I are indeed **fortunate**, however. We have available to us **confirmation** of Dr. Sarno's theories in the form of **physical evidence**. Esther Sternberg, M.D. (Booklet #1 above) has documented it in her beautifully written book, "*The Balance Within*." Just listen to her *bona fides*. She is Director of the Molecular, Cellular, and Behavioral Integrative Neuroscience Program and Chief of the Section on Neuroendocrine Immunology and Behavior at the National Institute of Mental Health and National Institutes of Health. Despite Dr. Sternberg's difficulty in printing her title on her business card, we **owe her a careful listen**. Take another look at the section on her book in Booklet #1 on Diet.

If you have been diagnosed with **any** of the following, this information on **TMS** is **relevant to you**: back, neck or shoulder pain; slipped disc; heartburn; hiatus hernia; ulcers; peptic ulcers; irritable bowel syndrome; spastic colon; constipation; gas; fibromyalgia; allergic rhinitis (hay fever); shingles; rheumatoid arthritis; bursitis; diabetes; lupus erythematosus; multiple sclerosis; heart palpitations; mitral valve prolapse; and arteriosclerosis.

Take Dr. Sarno's book to bed with you. **Read it with an open mind**. Get up determined to do all you can to overcome the **mental/emotional** component of your "disease." I'm not belittling the seriousness of your condition. I'm only urging you to try the technique that has worked for **so many other patients** without the need for chemicals, with all their **expense and side effects**.

Be well and God Bless You!

INDEX

Kinsolving, Dr. Richard, xv, 85, 173
Koch, Dr. William, 27
Krebiozen, 27

L

Lab One, 74
Laetrile, 182, 183, 184, 185, 186, 187, 188, 189, 247
Lai, Harry, 162
Laibow, Dr. Rima, 259
Lane Labs, 17, 18, 89, 189, 190, 193
Lanigan, A.J., 85
Las Mariposas Clinic, 180
Leukemia, x, 65, 108, 163
Levin, M.D., Alan, 210, 242
Ley, Dr. Herbert, 30
Life Extension, xv, 12, 66, 83, 256
Lipids, 217
Live Blood Cell Analysis, 75
Livingston, M.D., Virginia, 217, 225
Los Angeles Times, 22, 24, 38
Lynes, Barry, 239, 240, 241, 247

M

MacWilliam, Lyle, 57
Magnetic Therapy, 196
Mason, Roger, xv, 164
McCabe, Ed, 100
McClam. Erin, 289
McGill Cancer Center, 38
McLaughlin, Dr. Jerry, 152, 153
Merck, 19, 35

Mercola, Dr. Joseph, xv, 29, 31
Metastasis, 109
Mexican cancer clinics, 178
MGN-3, vi, ix, 17, 88, 89, 90, 91, 93, 189, 214, 224
Molinari, Congressman Guy, 219
Monoclonal antibodies, 224
Mountain Home Nutritionals, 57, 125
Moye, Dr. Lemuel, 23
Moyers, Bill, 209

N

Naessens, Gaston, 27, 216, 217
National Foundation for Alternative Medicine, 13
Natural Cancer Treatments That Work, 229, 230
Natural Killer Cell Activity Test, 77, 78
Natural Solutions Foundation, 89, 259
Nauts, D.Sc., Helen Coley, 225
Navarro Clinic, 135, 136, 138, 186
Navarro, Dr. Efren, 136, 138
Nelson, Dr. Brad, 129
New England Journal of Medicine, 24, 66
New Hope Medical Center, 174
Nieper, Dr. Hans, 187
Nolvadex, 20
Null, Gary, 250

Y

Young, Robert O., 116

Z

Zoladex, 20
Zubrod, Dr. Gordon, 65

ARCADIA PUBLIC LIBRARY
ARCADIA, WI 54612

CPSIA information can be obtained at www.ICGtesting.com
227814LV00002B/27/P